CGRN
Exam
SECRETS

Study Guide
Your Key to Exam Success

CGRN Test Review for the
American Board of Certification
for Gastroenterology Nurses
(ABCGN) RN Examination

Dear Future Exam Success Story:

First of all, **THANK YOU** for purchasing Mometrix study materials!

Second, congratulations! You are one of the few determined test-takers who are committed to doing whatever it takes to excel on your exam. **You have come to the right place.** We developed these study materials with one goal in mind: to deliver you the information you need in a format that's concise and easy to use.

In addition to optimizing your guide for the content of the test, we've outlined our recommended steps for breaking down the preparation process into small, attainable goals so you can make sure you stay on track.

We've also analyzed the entire test-taking process, identifying the most common pitfalls and showing how you can overcome them and be ready for any curveball the test throws you.

Standardized testing is one of the biggest obstacles on your road to success, which only increases the importance of doing well in the high-pressure, high-stakes environment of test day. Your results on this test could have a significant impact on your future, and this guide provides the information and practical advice to help you achieve your full potential on test day.

Your success is our success

We would love to hear from you! If you would like to share the story of your exam success or if you have any questions or comments in regard to our products, please contact us at **800-673-8175** or **support@mometrix.com**.

Thanks again for your business and we wish you continued success!

Sincerely,
The Mometrix Test Preparation Team

Need more help? Check out our flashcards at: http://mometrixflashcards.com/CGRN

TABLE OF CONTENTS

Introduction

Thank you for purchasing this resource! You have made the choice to prepare yourself for a test that could have a huge impact on your future, and this guide is designed to help you be fully ready for test day. Obviously, it's important to have a solid understanding of the test material, but you also need to be prepared for the unique environment and stressors of the test, so that you can perform to the best of your abilities.

For this purpose, the first section that appears in this guide is the **Secret Keys**. We've devoted countless hours to meticulously researching what works and what doesn't, and we've boiled down our findings to the five most impactful steps you can take to improve your performance on the test. We start at the beginning with study planning and move through the preparation process, all the way to the testing strategies that will help you get the most out of what you know when you're finally sitting in front of the test.

We recommend that you start preparing for your test as far in advance as possible. However, if you've bought this guide as a last-minute study resource and only have a few days before your test, we recommend that you skip over the first two Secret Keys since they address a long-term study plan.

If you struggle with **test anxiety**, we strongly encourage you to check out our recommendations for how you can overcome it. Test anxiety is a formidable foe, but it can be beaten, and we want to make sure you have the tools you need to defeat it.

Secret Key #1 – Plan Big, Study Small

There's a lot riding on your performance. If you want to ace this test, you're going to need to keep your skills sharp and the material fresh in your mind. You need a plan that lets you review everything you need to know while still fitting in your schedule. We'll break this strategy down into three categories.

Information Organization

Start with the information you already have: the official test outline. From this, you can make a complete list of all the concepts you need to cover before the test. Organize these concepts into groups that can be studied together, and create a list of any related vocabulary you need to learn so you can brush up on any difficult terms. You'll want to keep this vocabulary list handy once you actually start studying since you may need to add to it along the way.

Time Management

Once you have your set of study concepts, decide how to spread them out over the time you have left before the test. Break your study plan into small, clear goals so you have a manageable task for each day and know exactly what you're doing. Then just focus on one small step at a time. When you manage your time this way, you don't need to spend hours at a time studying. Studying a small block of content for a short period each day helps you retain information better and avoid stressing over how much you have left to do. You can relax knowing that you have a plan to cover everything in time. In order for this strategy to be effective though, you have to start studying early and stick to your schedule. Avoid the exhaustion and futility that comes from last-minute cramming!

Study Environment

The environment you study in has a big impact on your learning. Studying in a coffee shop, while probably more enjoyable, is not likely to be as fruitful as studying in a quiet room. It's important to keep distractions to a minimum. You're only planning to study for a short block of time, so make the most of it. Don't pause to check your phone or get up to find a snack. It's also important to **avoid multitasking**. Research has consistently shown that multitasking will make your studying dramatically less effective. Your study area should also be comfortable and well-lit so you don't have the distraction of straining your eyes or sitting on an uncomfortable chair.

The time of day you study is also important. You want to be rested and alert. Don't wait until just before bedtime. Study when you'll be most likely to comprehend and remember. Even better, if you know what time of day your test will be, set that time aside for study. That way your brain will be used to working on that subject at that specific time and you'll have a better chance of recalling information.

Finally, it can be helpful to team up with others who are studying for the same test. Your actual studying should be done in as isolated an environment as possible, but the work of organizing the information and setting up the study plan can be divided up. In between study sessions, you can discuss with your teammates the concepts that you're all studying and quiz each other on the details. Just be sure that your teammates are as serious about the test as you are. If you find that your study time is being replaced with social time, you might need to find a new team.

Secret Key #2 – Make Your Studying Count

You're devoting a lot of time and effort to preparing for this test, so you want to be absolutely certain it will pay off. This means doing more than just reading the content and hoping you can remember it on test day. It's important to make every minute of study count. There are two main areas you can focus on to make your studying count:

Retention

It doesn't matter how much time you study if you can't remember the material. You need to make sure you are retaining the concepts. To check your retention of the information you're learning, try recalling it at later times with minimal prompting. Try carrying around flashcards and glance at one or two from time to time or ask a friend who's also studying for the test to quiz you.

To enhance your retention, look for ways to put the information into practice so that you can apply it rather than simply recalling it. If you're using the information in practical ways, it will be much easier to remember. Similarly, it helps to solidify a concept in your mind if you're not only reading it to yourself but also explaining it to someone else. Ask a friend to let you teach them about a concept you're a little shaky on (or speak aloud to an imaginary audience if necessary). As you try to summarize, define, give examples, and answer your friend's questions, you'll understand the concepts better and they will stay with you longer. Finally, step back for a big picture view and ask yourself how each piece of information fits with the whole subject. When you link the different concepts together and see them working together as a whole, it's easier to remember the individual components.

Finally, practice showing your work on any multi-step problems, even if you're just studying. Writing out each step you take to solve a problem will help solidify the process in your mind, and you'll be more likely to remember it during the test.

Modality

Modality simply refers to the means or method by which you study. Choosing a study modality that fits your own individual learning style is crucial. No two people learn best in exactly the same way, so it's important to know your strengths and use them to your advantage.

For example, if you learn best by visualization, focus on visualizing a concept in your mind and draw an image or a diagram. Try color-coding your notes, illustrating them, or creating symbols that will trigger your mind to recall a learned concept. If you learn best by hearing or discussing information, find a study partner who learns the same way or read aloud to yourself. Think about how to put the information in your own words. Imagine that you are giving a lecture on the topic and record yourself so you can listen to it later.

For any learning style, flashcards can be helpful. Organize the information so you can take advantage of spare moments to review. Underline key words or phrases. Use different colors for different categories. Mnemonic devices (such as creating a short list in which every item starts with the same letter) can also help with retention. Find what works best for you and use it to store the information in your mind most effectively and easily.

Secret Key #3 – Practice the Right Way

Your success on test day depends not only on how many hours you put into preparing, but also on whether you prepared the right way. It's good to check along the way to see if your studying is paying off. One of the most effective ways to do this is by taking practice tests to evaluate your progress. Practice tests are useful because they show exactly where you need to improve. Every time you take a practice test, pay special attention to these three groups of questions:

- The questions you got wrong
- The questions you had to guess on, even if you guessed right
- The questions you found difficult or slow to work through

This will show you exactly what your weak areas are, and where you need to devote more study time. Ask yourself why each of these questions gave you trouble. Was it because you didn't understand the material? Was it because you didn't remember the vocabulary? Do you need more repetitions on this type of question to build speed and confidence? Dig into those questions and figure out how you can strengthen your weak areas as you go back to review the material.

Additionally, many practice tests have a section explaining the answer choices. It can be tempting to read the explanation and think that you now have a good understanding of the concept. However, an explanation likely only covers part of the question's broader context. Even if the explanation makes sense, **go back and investigate** every concept related to the question until you're positive you have a thorough understanding.

As you go along, keep in mind that the practice test is just that: practice. Memorizing these questions and answers will not be very helpful on the actual test because it is unlikely to have any of the same exact questions. If you only know the right answers to the sample questions, you won't be prepared for the real thing. **Study the concepts** until you understand them fully, and then you'll be able to answer any question that shows up on the test.

It's important to wait on the practice tests until you're ready. If you take a test on your first day of study, you may be overwhelmed by the amount of material covered and how much you need to learn. Work up to it gradually.

On test day, you'll need to be prepared for answering questions, managing your time, and using the test-taking strategies you've learned. It's a lot to balance, like a mental marathon that will have a big impact on your future. Like training for a marathon, you'll need to start slowly and work your way up. When test day arrives, you'll be ready.

Start with the strategies you've read in the first two Secret Keys—plan your course and study in the way that works best for you. If you have time, consider using multiple study resources to get different approaches to the same concepts. It can be helpful to see difficult concepts from more than one angle. Then find a good source for practice tests. Many times, the test website will suggest potential study resources or provide sample tests.

Practice Test Strategy

When you're ready to start taking practice tests, follow this strategy:

Untimed and Open-Book Practice

Take the first test with no time constraints and with your notes and study guide handy. Take your time and focus on applying the strategies you've learned.

Timed and Open-Book Practice

Take the second practice test open-book as well, but set a timer and practice pacing yourself to finish in time.

Timed and Closed-Book Practice

Take any other practice tests as if it were test day. Set a timer and put away your study materials. Sit at a table or desk in a quiet room, imagine yourself at the testing center, and answer questions as quickly and accurately as possible.

Keep repeating timed and closed-book tests on a regular basis until you run out of practice tests or it's time for the actual test. Your mind will be ready for the schedule and stress of test day, and you'll be able to focus on recalling the material you've learned.

Secret Key #4 – Pace Yourself

Once you're fully prepared for the material on the test, your biggest challenge on test day will be managing your time. Just knowing that the clock is ticking can make you panic even if you have plenty of time left. Work on pacing yourself so you can build confidence against the time constraints of the exam. Pacing is a difficult skill to master, especially in a high-pressure environment, so **practice is vital**.

Set time expectations for your pace based on how much time is available. For example, if a section has 60 questions and the time limit is 30 minutes, you know you have to average 30 seconds or less per question in order to answer them all. Although 30 seconds is the hard limit, set 25 seconds per question as your goal, so you reserve extra time to spend on harder questions. When you budget extra time for the harder questions, you no longer have any reason to stress when those questions take longer to answer.

Don't let this time expectation distract you from working through the test at a calm, steady pace, but keep it in mind so you don't spend too much time on any one question. Recognize that taking extra time on one question you don't understand may keep you from answering two that you do understand later in the test. If your time limit for a question is up and you're still not sure of the answer, mark it and move on, and come back to it later if the time and the test format allow. If the testing format doesn't allow you to return to earlier questions, just make an educated guess; then put it out of your mind and move on.

On the easier questions, be careful not to rush. It may seem wise to hurry through them so you have more time for the challenging ones, but it's not worth missing one if you know the concept and just didn't take the time to read the question fully. Work efficiently but make sure you understand the question and have looked at all of the answer choices, since more than one may seem right at first.

Even if you're paying attention to the time, you may find yourself a little behind at some point. You should speed up to get back on track, but do so wisely. Don't panic; just take a few seconds less on each question until you're caught up. Don't guess without thinking, but do look through the answer choices and eliminate any you know are wrong. If you can get down to two choices, it is often worthwhile to guess from those. Once you've chosen an answer, move on and don't dwell on any that you skipped or had to hurry through. If a question was taking too long, chances are it was one of the harder ones, so you weren't as likely to get it right anyway.

On the other hand, if you find yourself getting ahead of schedule, it may be beneficial to slow down a little. The more quickly you work, the more likely you are to make a careless mistake that will affect your score. You've budgeted time for each question, so don't be afraid to spend that time. Practice an efficient but careful pace to get the most out of the time you have.

Secret Key #5 – Have a Plan for Guessing

When you're taking the test, you may find yourself stuck on a question. Some of the answer choices seem better than others, but you don't see the one answer choice that is obviously correct. What do you do?

The scenario described above is very common, yet most test takers have not effectively prepared for it. Developing and practicing a plan for guessing may be one of the single most effective uses of your time as you get ready for the exam.

In developing your plan for guessing, there are three questions to address:

- When should you start the guessing process?
- How should you narrow down the choices?
- Which answer should you choose?

When to Start the Guessing Process

Unless your plan for guessing is to select C every time (which, despite its merits, is not what we recommend), you need to leave yourself enough time to apply your answer elimination strategies. Since you have a limited amount of time for each question, that means that if you're going to give yourself the best shot at guessing correctly, you have to decide quickly whether or not you will guess.

Of course, the best-case scenario is that you don't have to guess at all, so first, see if you can answer the question based on your knowledge of the subject and basic reasoning skills. Focus on the key words in the question and try to jog your memory of related topics. Give yourself a chance to bring the knowledge to mind, but once you realize that you don't have (or you can't access) the knowledge you need to answer the question, it's time to start the guessing process.

It's almost always better to start the guessing process too early than too late. It only takes a few seconds to remember something and answer the question from knowledge. Carefully eliminating wrong answer choices takes longer. Plus, going through the process of eliminating answer choices can actually help jog your memory.

Summary: Start the guessing process as soon as you decide that you can't answer the question based on your knowledge.

- 7 -

How to Narrow Down the Choices

The next chapter in this book (**Test-Taking Strategies**) includes a wide range of strategies for how to approach questions and how to look for answer choices to eliminate. You will definitely want to read those carefully, practice them, and figure out which ones work best for you. Here though, we're going to address a mindset rather than a particular strategy.

Your chances of guessing an answer correctly depend on how many options you are choosing from.

How many choices you have	How likely you are to guess correctly
5	20%
4	25%
3	33%
2	50%
1	100%

You can see from this chart just how valuable it is to be able to eliminate incorrect answers and make an educated guess, but there are two things that many test takers do that cause them to miss out on the benefits of guessing:

- Accidentally eliminating the correct answer
- Selecting an answer based on an impression

We'll look at the first one here, and the second one in the next section.

To avoid accidentally eliminating the correct answer, we recommend a thought exercise called **the $5 challenge**. In this challenge, you only eliminate an answer choice from contention if you are willing to bet $5 on it being wrong. Why $5? Five dollars is a small but not insignificant amount of money. It's an amount you could afford to lose but wouldn't want to throw away. And while losing $5 once might not hurt too much, doing it twenty times will set you back $100. In the same way, each small decision you make—eliminating a choice here, guessing on a question there—won't by itself impact your score very much, but when you put them all together, they can make a big difference. By holding each answer choice elimination decision to a higher standard, you can reduce the risk of accidentally eliminating the correct answer.

The $5 challenge can also be applied in a positive sense: If you are willing to bet $5 that an answer choice *is* correct, go ahead and mark it as correct.

Summary: Only eliminate an answer choice if you are willing to bet $5 that it is wrong.

Which Answer to Choose

You're taking the test. You've run into a hard question and decided you'll have to guess. You've eliminated all the answer choices you're willing to bet $5 on. Now you have to pick an answer. Why do we even need to talk about this? Why can't you just pick whichever one you feel like when the time comes?

The answer to these questions is that if you don't come into the test with a plan, you'll rely on your impression to select an answer choice, and if you do that, you risk falling into a trap. The test writers know that everyone who takes their test will be guessing on some of the questions, so they intentionally write wrong answer choices to seem plausible. You still have to pick an answer though, and if the wrong answer choices are designed to look right, how can you ever be sure that you're not falling for their trap? The best solution we've found to this dilemma is to take the decision out of your hands entirely. Here is the process we recommend:

Once you've eliminated any choices that you are confident (willing to bet $5) are wrong, select the first remaining choice as your answer.

Whether you choose to select the first remaining choice, the second, or the last, the important thing is that you use some preselected standard. Using this approach guarantees that you will not be enticed into selecting an answer choice that looks right, because you are not basing your decision on how the answer choices look.

This is not meant to make you question your knowledge. Instead, it is to help you recognize the difference between your knowledge and your impressions. There's a huge difference between thinking an answer is right because of what you know, and thinking an answer is right because it looks or sounds like it should be right.

Summary: To ensure that your selection is appropriately random, make a predetermined selection from among all answer choices you have not eliminated.

Test-Taking Strategies

This section contains a list of test-taking strategies that you may find helpful as you work through the test. By taking what you know and applying logical thought, you can maximize your chances of answering any question correctly!

It is very important to realize that every question is different and every person is different: no single strategy will work on every question, and no single strategy will work for every person. That's why we've included all of them here, so you can try them out and determine which ones work best for different types of questions and which ones work best for you.

Question Strategies

Read Carefully

Read the question and answer choices carefully. Don't miss the question because you misread the terms. You have plenty of time to read each question thoroughly and make sure you understand what is being asked. Yet a happy medium must be attained, so don't waste too much time. You must read carefully, but efficiently.

Contextual Clues

Look for contextual clues. If the question includes a word you are not familiar with, look at the immediate context for some indication of what the word might mean. Contextual clues can often give you all the information you need to decipher the meaning of an unfamiliar word. Even if you can't determine the meaning, you may be able to narrow down the possibilities enough to make a solid guess at the answer to the question.

Prefixes

If you're having trouble with a word in the question or answer choices, try dissecting it. Take advantage of every clue that the word might include. Prefixes and suffixes can be a huge help. Usually they allow you to determine a basic meaning. Pre- means before, post- means after, pro - is positive, de- is negative. From prefixes and suffixes, you can get an idea of the general meaning of the word and try to put it into context.

Hedge Words

Watch out for critical hedge words, such as *likely, may, can, sometimes, often, almost, mostly, usually, generally, rarely*, and *sometimes*. Question writers insert these hedge phrases to cover every possibility. Often an answer choice will be wrong simply because it leaves no room for exception. Be on guard for answer choices that have definitive words such as *exactly* and *always*.

Switchback Words

Stay alert for *switchbacks*. These are the words and phrases frequently used to alert you to shifts in thought. The most common switchback words are *but, although*, and *however*. Others include *nevertheless, on the other hand, even though, while, in spite of, despite, regardless of*. Switchback words are important to catch because they can change the direction of the question or an answer choice.

Face Value

When in doubt, use common sense. Accept the situation in the problem at face value. Don't read too much into it. These problems will not require you to make wild assumptions. If you have to go beyond creativity and warp time or space in order to have an answer choice fit the question, then you should move on and consider the other answer choices. These are normal problems rooted in reality. The applicable relationship or explanation may not be readily apparent, but it is there for you to figure out. Use your common sense to interpret anything that isn't clear.

Answer Choice Strategies

Answer Selection

The most thorough way to pick an answer choice is to identify and eliminate wrong answers until only one is left, then confirm it is the correct answer. Sometimes an answer choice may immediately seem right, but be careful. The test writers will usually put more than one reasonable answer choice on each question, so take a second to read all of them and make sure that the other choices are not equally obvious. As long as you have time left, it is better to read every answer choice than to pick the first one that looks right without checking the others.

Answer Choice Families

An answer choice family consists of two (in rare cases, three) answer choices that are very similar in construction and cannot all be true at the same time. If you see two answer choices that are direct opposites or parallels, one of them is usually the correct answer. For instance, if one answer choice says that quantity x increases and another either says that quantity x decreases (opposite) or says that quantity y increases (parallel), then those answer choices would fall into the same family. An answer choice that doesn't match the construction of the answer choice family is more likely to be incorrect. Most questions will not have answer choice families, but when they do appear, you should be prepared to recognize them.

Eliminate Answers

Eliminate answer choices as soon as you realize they are wrong, but make sure you consider all possibilities. If you are eliminating answer choices and realize that the last one you are left with is also wrong, don't panic. Start over and consider each choice again. There may be something you missed the first time that you will realize on the second pass.

Avoid Fact Traps

Don't be distracted by an answer choice that is factually true but doesn't answer the question. You are looking for the choice that answers the question. Stay focused on what the question is asking for so you don't accidentally pick an answer that is true but incorrect. Always go back to the question and make sure the answer choice you've selected actually answers the question and is not merely a true statement.

Extreme Statements

In general, you should avoid answers that put forth extreme actions as standard practice or proclaim controversial ideas as established fact. An answer choice that states the "process should be used in certain situations, if..." is much more likely to be correct than one that states the "process should be discontinued completely." The first is a calm rational statement and doesn't even make a definitive, uncompromising stance, using a hedge word *if* to provide wiggle room, whereas the second choice is a radical idea and far more extreme.

Benchmark

As you read through the answer choices and you come across one that seems to answer the question well, mentally select that answer choice. This is not your final answer, but it's the one that will help you evaluate the other answer choices. The one that you selected is your benchmark or standard for judging each of the other answer choices. Every other answer choice must be compared to your benchmark. That choice is correct until proven otherwise by another answer choice beating it. If you find a better answer, then that one becomes your new benchmark. Once you've decided that no other choice answers the question as well as your benchmark, you have your final answer.

Predict the Answer

Before you even start looking at the answer choices, it is often best to try to predict the answer. When you come up with the answer on your own, it is easier to avoid distractions and traps because you will know exactly what to look for. The right answer choice is unlikely to be word-for-word what you came up with, but it should be a close match. Even if you are confident that you have the right answer, you should still take the time to read each option before moving on.

General Strategies

Tough Questions

If you are stumped on a problem or it appears too hard or too difficult, don't waste time. Move on! Remember though, if you can quickly check for obviously incorrect answer choices, your chances of guessing correctly are greatly improved. Before you completely give up, at least try to knock out a couple of possible answers. Eliminate what you can and then guess at the remaining answer choices before moving on.

Check Your Work

Since you will probably not know every term listed and the answer to every question, it is important that you get credit for the ones that you do know. Don't miss any questions through careless mistakes. If at all possible, try to take a second to look back over your answer selection and make sure you've selected the correct answer choice and haven't made a costly careless mistake (such as marking an answer choice that you didn't mean to mark). This quick double check should more than pay for itself in caught mistakes for the time it costs.

Pace Yourself

It's easy to be overwhelmed when you're looking at a page full of questions; your mind is confused and full of random thoughts, and the clock is ticking down faster than you would like. Calm down and maintain the pace that you have set for yourself. Especially as you get down to the last few minutes of the test, don't let the small numbers on the clock make you panic. As long as you are on track by monitoring your pace, you are guaranteed to have time for each question.

Don't Rush

It is very easy to make errors when you are in a hurry. Maintaining a fast pace in answering questions is pointless if it makes you miss questions that you would have gotten right otherwise. Test writers like to include distracting information and wrong answers that seem right. Taking a little extra time to avoid careless mistakes can make all the difference in your test score. Find a pace that allows you to be confident in the answers that you select.

Keep Moving

Panicking will not help you pass the test, so do your best to stay calm and keep moving. Taking deep breaths and going through the answer elimination steps you practiced can help to break through a stress barrier and keep your pace.

Final Notes

The combination of a solid foundation of content knowledge and the confidence that comes from practicing your plan for applying that knowledge is the key to maximizing your performance on test day. As your foundation of content knowledge is built up and strengthened, you'll find that the strategies included in this chapter become more and more effective in helping you quickly sift through the distractions and traps of the test to isolate the correct answer.

Now it's time to move on to the test content chapters of this book, but be sure to keep your goal in mind. As you read, think about how you will be able to apply this information on the test. If you've already seen sample questions for the test and you have an idea of the question format and style, try to come up with questions of your own that you can answer based on what you're reading. This will give you valuable practice applying your knowledge in the same ways you can expect to on test day.

Good luck and good studying!

General Nursing Care

Development of Gastroenterology Nursing Field

The practice of nursing has been in existence for centuries. As medicine has advanced, so has nursing. This has led to specialization; health care providers direct their practice to treating one organ system. **Gastroenterology nursing** has become specialized, in parallel with the field of gastroenterology. With the introduction of a semiflexible scope by Rudolf Schindler, the gastroenterology field has grown tremendously. The need for nurses trained in the field has also mushroomed, ultimately leading to the practice of gastroenterology nursing. To develop standards of practice and goals for the gastroenterology nursing field, the Society of Gastrointestinal Assistants was formed in 1974. That group evolved into the Society of Gastroenterology Nurses and Associates, Inc. or SGNA.

Managing the Gastroenterology Department

There are five functions involved in **managing the gastroenterology department:** planning, organizing, directing, controlling and staffing. The manager of the gastroenterology department must consider resources, budgets, personnel and educational goals for the unit. The manager should confer with the staff in formulating any plans. Additionally, the manager must make informed decisions. Organizational practices can vary. The goal is to foster effective operations in the gastroenterology department. The manager should then direct the unit to accomplish the goals set by motivating and leading the staff. Control measures are established to foster the continued efficacy of the program. This entails setting clear standards, evaluating the process for efficacy, instituting improvements where needed, and staffing the unit.

Responsibilities of Gastroenterology Nurse

The SGNA is responsible for outlining the **practice and standards of gastroenterology nursing.** This organization establishes standards that should be practiced to provide adequate care for the patient. The care givers must address patient needs first. Nurses must ascertain medical history, comfort levels, psychological concerns and educational needs. During any treatment or intervention, the patient must be monitored for safety and comfort. During follow up, the patient needs to be monitored for appropriate response and recovery. The gastroenterology nurse must be familiar with all equipment used. They need to be able to evaluate the instrument for problems, to assist in diagnostic or therapeutic Documentation of events, medications and outcomes need to be done. Maintaining and sharing knowledge is the responsibility of all members of the gastroenterology team.

Standards

SGNA has established **standards** for the outcome of the practice of gastroenterology nursing. Standards offer guides to assess practice and outcomes in the field. The standards addressed are quality of care, performance appraisal, education, collegiality, ethics, collaboration, research, and resource utilization. The Joint Commission has also established standards to ensure safety and quality. For a department to be certified by the Joint Commission, the department must demonstrate its ability to meet Joint Commission standards, such as infection control. Other standards must be met, as well. Different regulatory agencies demand that certain specifics be met to ensure the safety of patients and of personnel. These agencies include the Centers for Disease

Control and Prevention, the Environmental Protection Agency, the Food and Drug Administration, and the Occupational Safety and Health Administration.

Research Process

Gastroenterology nursing research allows for improving outcomes, procedures and practices in gastroenterology nursing. Once a problem or question has surfaced, the research process can be employed for a solution. This entails reviewing the knowledge available via literature and studies, formulating a hypothesis, setting up a study protocol, establishing measurement criteria for the data, collecting the data, analyzing the data and sharing conclusions.

Elements of Research

The following are **elements of research**:

- **Variable** is an entity that can be different within a population.
- **Independent variable** is the variable that the researchers change to evaluate its effect.
- **Dependent variable** is the variable that may be changed by alterations in the independent variable.
- **Hypothesis** is the proposed explanation to describe an expected outcome in a study.
- **Sample** is the selected population to be studied.
- **The experimental group** is that population within the sample that undergoes the treatment or intervention.
- **The control group** is that population within the sample that is not exposed to the treatment of intervention being evaluated.

Purpose of Nursing Assessment

Nursing assessment evaluates patient data to help in diagnosis and treatment. The nurse assesses baseline health and medical history to be sure the patient will be safe. The nurse also determines what limitations the patient may have in terms of understanding or cooperation. Nursing assessment is an ongoing process, which includes baseline information, information on the patient's response and recovery to the intervention and continued efforts to maintain the patient's health. The nurse can collaborate with other team members to help in this assessment.

Purpose of Nursing Diagnosis and Planning

Nursing diagnosis is directed at patient comfort and outcome. Nurses establish nursing interventions that are needed for the patient to be safe and comfortable. The nurse uses the diagnosis to direct therapies and to anticipate potentially needed interventions. **Planning** allows the nurse to outline the methods needed to achieve patient goals. This accounts for alternative therapies that may be needed, setting priorities, satisfactory outcomes to be achieved, and expectations for discharge. The gastroenterology nurse needs to document the plan. The plan outlines nursing responsibilities, possible interventions, and expected outcomes.

Implementation of Nursing Plan

Implementing the nursing plan requires a measure of fluidity. The original plan is based on initial data. As new data is accumulated, however, the original plan may be modified. There is a need to incorporate individual needs of the patient as the plan proceeds. Different interventions may be called for depending on individual responses or limitations. The nurse needs to continually monitor the patient's response and status to be able to offer appropriate nursing interventions.

Documentation is essential at every step of the way. The information can be useful in further treatment of the individual. It can also be used to assess the process so that improvements or adjustments can be made. The documentation may also be used for research purposes to further the knowledge of gastroenterology practice. The record may become necessary for legal purposes, as well.

Evaluation Process

In order to provide the best care for the patient, the nurse must **evaluate** the process in effect. This entails reviewing procedures and interventions in relation to standards of care, quality of care, and patient outcomes. Critical evaluation of the nursing process can lead to changes that may improve the quality of care for patients and/or identify personnel issues that need to be addressed. Modifying care plans is important to maintaining effective patient care. Deficiencies may be noted and can, therefore, be addressed. This underscores the importance of adequate documentation. In order to evaluate the process, the nurse must have access to the documentation to assess the present process. This evaluation may lead to changes that improve the quality of care in the gastroenterology department.

Health Status Through Data Collection

Assessment of Cultural Elements of Wellness

A **cultural assessment** can begin by asking the patient with which cultural group the patient most identifies and by careful observation of patient responses and interactions. The Giger and Davidhizar's Transcultural Assessment Model can serve as a guide. Elements include:

- *Cultural*: The country in which the person was born; their ethnicity; how long the person has lived in this country if born outside of the United States.
- *Biologic*: Color of skin and hair, body structure, ethnic-specific disorders, dietary preferences, psychological characteristics.
- *Environmental*: Cultural health practices and values, perceptions of health/sickness.
- *Time*: Perceptions of time, work and social time. Past (focus on maintaining traditions), present (focus on here and now, avoids planning), or future orientation (focus on future goals).
- *Social*: Roles of culture, family, ethnicity, religion, work, friends, types of leisure activities.
- *Spatial*: Proxemics, body language.
- *Communicative*: Language abilities and preferences, voice quality, non-verbal language (gestures, eye contact), pronunciation/enunciation.

Assessment of Psychosocial Elements of Wellness

A **psychosocial assessment** should provide additional information to the physical assessment to guide the patient's plan of care and should include:

- Previous hospitalizations and experience with healthcare.
- Psychiatric history: Suicidal ideation, psychiatric disorders, family psychiatric history, history of violence and/or self-mutilation.
- Chief complaint: Patient's perception.
- Complementary therapies: Acupuncture, visualization, and meditation.
- Occupational and educational background: Employment, retirement, and special skills.
- Social patterns: Family and friends, living situation, typical activities, support system.

- Sexual patterns: Orientation, problems, and sex practices.
- Interests/abilities: Hobbies and sports.
- Current or past substance abuse: Type, frequency, drinking pattern, use of recreational drugs, and overuse of prescription drugs.
- Ability to cope: Stress reduction techniques.
- Physical, sexual, emotional, and financial abuse: Older adults are especially vulnerable to abuse and may be reluctant to disclose out of shame or fear.
- Spiritual/Cultural assessment: Religious/Spiritual importance, practices, restrictions (such as blood products or foods), and impact on health/health decisions.

Assessment of Spiritual Elements of Wellness

HOPE is a simple mnemonic used as a guideline for the spiritual assessment:

- **H**ope – What sources of hope (who or what) do you have to turn to?
- **O**rganized – Are you a part of an organized religion or faith group? What do you gain from membership in this group?
- **P**ersonal – What spiritual practices (prayer, meditation) are most helpful?
- **E**ffects – What effects do your beliefs play on any medical care or end-of-life issues and decisions? Do you have any beliefs that may affect the type of care the health care team can provide you with?

FICA is another abbreviated spiritual assessment tool:

- **F**aith - Do you have a faith or belief system that gives your life meaning?
- **I**mportance - What importance does your faith have in your daily life?
- **C**ommunity - Do you participate and gain support from a faith community?
- **A**ddress - What faith issues would you like me to address in your care?

Importance of Pharmacology Assessment Upon Patient Admission for Procedures

A **pharmacology assessment** is especially important upon patient admission for a procedure because some medications may interfere with testing and others may increase the risk of complications. Patients should be advised to bring all current medications with them for the procedure so they can be examined as patients are not always good reporters and may overlook some medications if simply asked to list them. Assessment should include questions about what the patient was advised to do about medications the day of the procedure and whether the patient followed those directions, what prescriptions, OTC, supplements, and herbal preparations the patient normally takes as well as their dosages and when the last dose of each was taken. The patient should also be asked about any allergies the patient has, especially to any drugs or to latex, and what type of adverse reactions the patient has experienced.

Impact of Medications on Gastroenterology Procedures

Some **medications, supplements, and herbal preparations** can impact gastroenterology procedures:

- *Prescription medications:* Blood thinners are of special concern because of increased risk of bleeding. For low-risk procedures, anti-platelet agents, warfarin, and novel oral anticoagulants are generally continued, but for high-risk procedures, medications may be withheld for 5 to 7 days prior to the procedure. Insulin is usually administered with a half-dosage prior to the procedure and half with a post-procedure meal. Oral antidiabetics agents are usually withheld the day of the procedure until after completion.
- *OTC medications:* Because of increased risk of bleeding and interference with visualization, aspirin products and Pepto-Bismol® are generally withheld for 7 days prior to GI procedures and NSAIDs for 5 days. Antacids are withheld the day of the procedure. All other OTC medications should be withheld for 5 days.
- *Supplements*: Preparations that include iron are usually withheld for 7 days prior to a procedure.
- *Herbals*: Gingko increases the risk of bleeding, especially if patients also take other blood-thinning drugs and should be discontinued for 5 to 7 days prior to a procedure.

GI Anatomy, Physiology, and Pathophysiology

Cross Section of the Esophagus

The **inner lining of the esophagus** is composed of squamous epithelium that abuts connective tissue called the lamina propria. The **middle layer or submucosa** consists of fibrous and connective tissue with nerves and blood vessels. It is separated from the lamina propria by a smooth muscle band called the muscularis mucosae. The **muscularis layer** is the outside tissue that has a layer of circular muscles followed by a layer of longitudinal muscle fibers. The Auerbach's nerve plexus lies between these muscle layers. At the **upper portion of the esophagus**, there is a small area of striated muscle. The lower half of the esophagus has smooth muscle. There is a transition from striated muscle, which accounts for the first 5% of esophageal muscle, to the approximately 50% distal end composed of smooth muscle.

GERD

Gastroesophageal reflux disease (**GERD**) is caused by reflux of gastric contents into the esophagus. Although some reflux is normal, when the reflux causes symptoms it is considered abnormal. The reflux of the acidic contents of the stomach into the esophagus causes an inflammatory reaction in the esophageal mucosa. Long term reflux can lead to Barrett's esophagus in which the normal mucosal cells are replaced by columnar epithelium. Patients complain of heartburn, dysphagia, and chest pain. Some may have coughing or wheezing if reflux contents are aspirated.

Diagnosis

Diagnosis of GERD can be made several ways.

- A *barium swallow* entails taking X-rays of swallowed barium as it passes through the esophagus. This can determine if there is an obstruction or other abnormality.
- *Endoscopy* can also be done, allowing for visualization of the lining of the esophagus, looking for abnormalities, masses, or inflammation. This procedure can also obtain a biopsy for tissue.

Other tests may be indicated.

- *Manometry* is a test to measure muscle coordination and esophageal pressures. This may help to diagnose a motility disorder.
- A *24-hour pH study* can determine the rate and time of reflux episodes and how these episodes may be related to other symptoms such as cough.
- Another test for correlating non-gastrointestinal symptoms with reflux is *gastric emptying studies*, which trace the path of a radioactive isotope that is swallowed by the patient.

Complications and Treatment

50% of GERD patients develop esophagitis. Other **complications** include stricture formation, esophageal ulcerations, Barrett's esophagus, gastrointestinal bleeding and aspiration pneumonia. To **treat** GERD, patients need to modify their diet to avoid things that may increase symptoms, such as coffee and alcohol. They must also attempt to lose weight if indicated. Other actions include avoiding lying down after eating for several hours and elevating the head during sleep. There are **medications** that may help with symptoms. These include antacids, H2 blockers, or proton pump inhibiters. Sometimes a motility agent is added to the regimen, such as bethanechol or raglan. For those refractory to treatment, surgery can be done.

Esophageal Cancer

Esophageal cancer is usually squamous cell in origin. There are a smaller number of adenocarcinomas that develop in individuals with Barrett's esophagus. Cancers of the esophagus are associated with chronic esophagitis, GERD, or tobacco and alcohol use. Patients present with dysphagia, odynophagia, weight loss and anorexia. **Diagnosis** can be made by esophagogastroduodenoscopy or EGD, which permits visualization and an opportunity for tissue biopsy. Patients also need to be evaluated for metastatic disease. **Treatment** is limited. Surgery can be done to alleviate symptoms. A stent can also be placed via EGD for obstructive symptoms. Despite treatment, the prognosis is poor, with a five-year survival rate of less than 5%.

Esophageal Varices

Causes and Symptoms

Esophageal varices are the result of portal hypertension due to cirrhosis or other diseases impinging on the portal circulation. Submucosal vessels in the distal part of the esophagus become enlarged because of increased pressure from the portal system. Varices may be asymptomatic, but they are at risk for sudden disruption and massive bleeding. This can be life-threatening, requiring emergency intervention. Patients may present with blood coming from the mouth, or they may be in hypovolemic shock. **Diagnosis** can be made endoscopically. All supportive measures need to be taken to care for the patient, including cardiovascular support and replacement of blood products.

Treatment of Bleeding Esophageal Varices

Treatment for esophageal varices depends on the clinical state of the patient. To manage acute situations, commonly esophageal sclerotherapy is performed. This entails use of an endoscope to inject sclerosing substances into the bleeding varices. Complications of this procedure include perforation, ulcerations and stricture formations. More recently, therapy for bleeding varices has included esophageal variceal ligation. Via the endoscope, bands are placed around the varices. Some esophageal variceal bleeding requires the use of esophageal tamponade. This is accomplished by introducing a balloon device to be inflated against the varices. **Preventive therapy** to reduce the risk of another bleeding episode calls for consideration of a portal venous shunt to relieve the pressure of the portal hypertension. This procedure is not suited to emergency situations, however, since it is a difficult procedure with high morbidity and mortality. A newer, non-surgical treatment is being favored, transjugular intrahepatic portosystemic shunt or TIPS.

Esophageal Strictures

Esophageal strictures, abnormal collections of fibrous tissue, can interfere with the passage of nutrients to the stomach. Strictures can be the result of infection, esophagitis, or caustic injuries. Patients commonly present with progressive dysphagia. **Treatment** requires reducing the stricture to relieve interference. The patient is treated by using different forms of dilators, such as balloons or plastics. This compresses the stricture, opening up the esophageal lumen. Often these patients will require repeat dilation procedures for recurrent symptoms. Children may require surgery because they often have strictures that are long. The most common complication of dilatation is perforation.

Removal of Foreign Bodies from the Esophagus

Esophageal foreign bodies may be acute or chronic. The nature of the foreign body dictates the treatment. Endoscopy using a snare can be employed to extract the object. If applicable, it can also be crushed so that it can pass into the stomach. Sometimes, in adults, medications can be used to relax the LES so that the substance can more easily continue into the stomach. Surgery must be considered for certain objects, such as illegal drugs or sharp objects. It also needs to be considered when there are complications like bleeding or perforation. Possible **complications** of ingested foreign objects include perforation, bleeding, or local irritation.

Caustic Injury to the Esophagus

Caustic injury can be caused by both alkaline and acidic toxins, but alkaline exposures are usually more harmful. Patients complain of pain and difficulty swallowing. **Diagnosis** requires evaluation for infection and/or perforation. An endoscopy is needed to assess the injury, but may be delayed since injuries may not appear immediately. Great care needs to be exercised to avoid perforation to the damaged area. **Treatment** varies, depending on the toxin. All patients must remain NPO, and a nasogastric tube should be placed. Subsequent complications may include strictures, which will need appropriate therapy. Some individuals are increased risk of cancer.

Infections of the Esophagus

Infections of the esophagus are much more likely to occur in people who are immunocompromised. The most common are *Candida*, herpes simplex, and cytomegalovirus or CMV. Patients present with dysphagia and odynophagia. With severe infection, nerves can be compromised leading to dysfunctional motility. Rarely, infection can result in perforation. Because these individuals suffer from underlying medical conditions that make them susceptible, the infections can become systemic. Definitive **diagnosis** requires endoscopy, which visualizes the mucosal surface and allows for tissue collection. With *Candida*, the first line of **treatment** is nystatin therapy. If infection persists or is severe, the patient can be given ketoconazole or amphotericin B. The viral infections are less likely to respond to curative treatment, but palliative treatment may help with symptoms.

Achalasia

Motility disorders cause disruption of the normal peristaltic motion of the esophagus, and may involve the LES. These disorders include achalasia, diffuse esophageal spasm and nutcracker

- 21 -

esophagus. **Achalasia** is the result of disrupted peristalsis and increased LES pressure. **Symptoms** of achalasia include dysphagia, regurgitation and weight loss. On Barium X-ray, the esophagus is dilated and ends sharply at the LES junction. **Treatment** includes eating slowly and concomitantly drinking fluids. Dilatation of the esophagus can be helpful. Some may need surgery, however. Those who are not surgical candidates can get some relief with nitrates or calcium channel blockers. Recently, there has been good success with injecting botulinum toxin into the LES. Long term, patients may suffer from esophagitis, aspiration pneumonia and an increased risk of cancer.

Barrett's Esophagus

Barrett's esophagus is the replacement of normal squamous epithelium by columnar epithelium. It is commonly associated with chronic reflux disease. **Symptoms** include those expected in reflux disease, such as heartburn, regurgitation and pain. **Diagnosis** requires an endoscopy to visualize the surface and obtain tissue. The reddish columnar epithelium can be seen jutting above the gastro-esophageal junction. **Treatment** is to relieve symptoms. The risk of cancer is increased in these patients. Therefore, the individual diagnosed with Barrett's esophagus should be regularly evaluated for progression of disease.

Stomach

The **stomach functions** to mix food with various substances and to move it to the small intestines for further processing. The digestion of proteins and fats begins in the stomach. As the stomach expands, the stomach muscles are stimulated to contract, causing stronger peristalsis. The stomach curves from the esophagus to the duodenum, where it joins the small intestines at the pyloric sphincter. The cardia is the initial portion, followed by the fundus, the body and the antrum. The antrum extends to the pylorus. The right curvature is called the lesser curvature; the left side is longer and is called the greater curvature.

Layers of Stomach Wall, Blood Supply, and Innervation

The **muscularis propria** is made of three muscles layers. These include the outer longitudinal muscle fibers, the middle circular smooth muscle and the inner transverse fiber layer. These muscles cause the peristalsis, which results in mixing the food. The next layer is the **submucosa**, which is mostly connective tissue with some blood vessels, some lymphatics and some nerves. The inner surface, or **gastric mucosa**, is covered with rugae, resembling wrinkles. This allows for the stomach to expand when contents enter from the esophagus. The blood supply of the stomach is drained through the **portal vein**. Arterial blood supply comes from the **celiac axis**. The **vagus nerve** provides parasympathetic innervation to the stomach, which stimulates secretion and motility. The sympathetic is responsible for pain, inhibition of secretion and of motility.

Gastric Glands Involved with Digestion

The stomach functions to begin the process of digestion. This requires the secretion of substances to help ready the food for the small intestines. There are **three glands** involved in this: the cardiac glands, the oxyntic glands, and the pyloric glands.

- *Cardiac glands* are located immediately after the transition to the stomach. They secrete mucous and pepsinogen, which then becomes pepsin when it reacts with hydrochloric acid.
- The *oxyntic glands*, which are contained in the upper 2/3 of the stomach, are composed of four different cells: chief cells, parietal cells, mucous neck cells and endocrine cells. Aside from secreting hydrochloric acid, the parietal cells secrete intrinsic factor, which allows for the absorption of the important vitamin B12.

- *Pyloric glands* are located in the antrum and pylorus areas of the stomach. Along with cells that secrete mucus and pepsinogen, these glands have the G cells for secreting gastrin.

Gastric Cancer

Gastric cancer is almost always adenocarcinoma. 3% are of other origins, including carcinoid tumors, lymphoma, leiomyosarcoma or sarcomas. Gastric cancer can be in a localized area, but it can also be of a diffuse nature. Diffuse cancer spreads through areas of the superficial layer of the gastric lining. Its occurrence can be associated with increasing age, male sex, family history and *Helicobacter pylori.* Patients present with pain, weight loss, vomiting, and occult blood. Cancers are commonly found in the antrum or the lesser curvature of the stomach. However, cancers related to gastric atrophy often affect the upper portion of the stomach.

Diagnosis and Treatment

X-rays can **diagnose** a lesion, but endoscopy is needed to obtain tissue for definitive diagnosis. Since gastric cancers can metastasize, an appropriate work up needs to be done to look for hematogenous, lymphatic or direct spread. The liver is the most common site for metastatic spread of gastric cancer. **Surgery** can be curative in some cases, requiring a partial gastrectomy. In this country, however, cancers are not usually diagnosed until the cancer is advanced. In those cases, surgery is for palliation. Surgery can relieve obstructive symptoms, manage bleeding or provide a method for adequate nutrition. Chemotherapy, radiation or a combination can be provided, but the prognosis is poor.

Gastric Varices

Gastric varices commonly occur in the upper part of the stomach. They result from the increased pressure due to portal hypertension. Diseases of the liver and portal circulation cause portal hypertension. Gastric varices are even more likely to cause death from gastrointestinal bleeding than are esophageal varices. **Diagnosis** is best accomplished with endoscopy. **Acute treatment** requires stabilizing the patient and treating the varices with tamponade via the Sengstaken-Blakemore tube or using octreotide. **Long term treatment** requires reducing the portal hypertension. This usually involves surgery to create a shunt for the portal circulation. The newer procedure of transjugular intrahepatic portosystemic shunt or TIPS is a less invasive way to reduce portal hypertension.

Hiatal Hernia

Hiatal hernia occurs when part of the stomach pushes through the diaphragm into the chest. Some of these hernias slide back and forth through the diaphragm. It is more likely to occur in the older patient and in women. This abnormality can result in decreased LES pressure and reflux. There is also a rolling hiatal hernia in which the greater curvature juts into the chest cavity, while the LES stays below the diaphragm. This is less common. Although these individuals complain of fullness, they do not suffer from reflux. **Diagnosis** can be made by routine Chest X-ray, Barium X-rays or endoscopy. **Treatment** requires weight loss, elevation of the head while sleeping, avoiding food for several hours before going to bed and medications such as H2 blockers and antacids.

Gastric Outlet Obstruction

Gastric outlet obstruction results when the passage of food is blocked from leaving the stomach. Patients present with vomiting, nausea, pain and symptoms of reflux. Some causes include masses, bezoars, polyps, and caustic exposures. Tests need to be conducted to determine outlet patency, such as radionuclide imaging. X-rays may also be useful. **Infants** are at risk of **hypertrophic pyloric stenosis**. The pyloric sphincter is dysfunctional, preventing food from leaving the stomach. These children have projectile vomiting and may suffer from dehydration and metabolic abnormalities. **Diagnosis** is accomplished by Barium X-rays. Treatment requires surgery, referred to as pyloromyotomy.

Bezoars

Bezoars are balls of hardened material that collect in the stomach. Some of these are composed of food matter known as phytobezoars. These are usually made up of plant or vegetable materials. These can be associated with such diseases as achlorhydria, decreased gastric motility, poorly chewed food and gastroparesis. Other bezoars can be composed of hair, and these are referred to as trichobezoars. This usually occurs in young women who chew their hair. It may be related to a psychiatric disorder. **Symptoms** include fullness, anorexia, vomiting, perforation or obstruction. Sometimes they result in irritation and ulceration of the mucosal surface. Clinicians can attempt to disrupt phytobezoars endoscopically. Surgery may be needed if this is unsuccessful. Trichobezoars require surgical removal.

Caustic Injury

Caustic injury to the stomach results from the ingestion of materials that damage the lining of the stomach. Both acid and alkaline substances can cause injury. It is more common for these substances to injure the more proximal gastrointestinal structures, but some individuals do suffer gastric injury. The exposure leads to ulceration, scarring and the risk of perforation. Patients need endoscopic examination to determine the extent of injury. Patients need to be evaluated for aspiration pneumonia or perforation. A common complication is stricture formation, which may require dilatation. Surgery may be required for severe scarring.

ZE Syndrome

Zollinger-Ellison (ZE) syndrome is a rare disease that causes tumors in the pancreas and duodenum. These tumors secrete gastrin, which causes the stomach to produce excess acid. This may lead to gastric and duodenal ulcers. The **symptoms** of this disease are those of peptic ulcer disease. Patients suffer from abdominal pain, nausea, vomiting, weight loss and bleeding. The **diagnosis** is made by measuring the level of gastrin in the blood. An endoscopy may be needed to check for gastric or duodenal ulcers. **Treatment** is directed towards reducing acid secretion in the stomach. The first line of therapy involves using proton-pump inhibitors such as omeprazole. Another option is use of the H-2 blockers like Cimetidine, but these are less effective. In general, however, these ulcers are less responsive to treatment than other ulcers. Surgery may be considered to remove the tumors and/or to treat the ulcers.

Nature of Gastritis

Gastritis is the result of an inflammation of the lining of the stomach. This condition can be acute or chronic. The inflammation is the result of an irritant, such as excess acid production, certain medications or bile exposure from the duodenum. The acute form of this disease can be related to acute illness, trauma, surgery or alcohol. Chronic gastritis may be associated with aging, *Helicobacter pylori,* cancer, pernicious anemia or ulcers. The inflammation can be superficial, involving the upper part of the lining. Atrophic gastritis, on the other hand, involves the full lining. Thus, there is atrophy of the gastric glands. With gastric atrophy, the lining is thinned with scant inflammation. There is loss of gastric glands. **Diagnosis** is best obtained by endoscopy. With chronic gastritis, there may be some bleeding that resolves spontaneously. Some patients develop a chronic anemia, however, with slow continual blood loss. **Treatment** is directed towards symptoms and complications, and may include H2 blockers, antacids, and sucralfate.

Peptic Ulcer Disease

Peptic ulcer disease is the most common cause of upper gastrointestinal bleeding. Peptic ulcers commonly present with abdominal pain, particularly pain that manifests while sleeping. Some people with ulcers are not aware of them until bleeding occurs. The mucosal lining of the gastrointestinal tract is disrupted, exposing the underlying tissue to damage from harmful substances. As the damage continues, blood vessels can be disturbed, leading to bleeding. In extreme cases, perforation can result.

Peptic ulcers result from a number of **causes**:

- Helicobacter pylori infection.
- Excessive exposure to certain drugs like non-steroidal anti-inflammatories.
- A history of ulcers in the family smoking.

The association of stress and ulcer formation is controversial.

Diagnosis and Complications

Although X-rays can reveal an ulcer, endoscopy is probably the preferred method for **diagnosis**. Endoscopic visualization detects smaller ulcers than X-rays. In addition, endoscopy allows for collection of tissue. This is particularly important for gastric ulcers, since they may be malignant. Ulcers commonly cause gastrointestinal hemorrhage. At times, this can be massive. Ulcers also lead to perforation, which may be further complicated by peritonitis. Some ulcers lead to penetration, meaning the ulcer penetrates into another abdominal organ, such as the liver or the colon. Depending on the location, ulcers can interfere with gastric emptying, causing motility problems.

Therapy

Treatment is tailored to the particular ulcer and associated complications. Although diet manipulation may be helpful in some individuals, medications are usually needed.

- *Proton pump inhibitors* interfere with the production of acid by inhibiting a necessary enzyme.
- *H2 blockers* interfere with histamine receptor sites on parietal cells. The action of these drugs reduces acid secretion.
- *Sucralfate* forms a barrier of protection in the damaged area, giving it insulation and time to heal.
- *Antacids* counter the acid produced in the stomach.
- *Cytotec, a prostaglandin,* offers protection because it opposes secretion of acid.

Treatment for a bleeding peptic ulcer requires the control of the bleeding, volume replacement to prevent or reverse shock, and treatment for the underlying cause of the disease. Complications from ulcer disease may need more invasive treatment, such as surgery.

Gastroparesis

Gastroparesis refers to a delayed emptying of stomach. Its cause is thought to be related to diabetic autonomic neuropathy. Gastric muscle activity is hypoactive or absent. Patients present with nausea, vomiting, abdominal distention, fullness, heartburn, abdominal pain or constipation.

Diagnosis is accomplished by radiologic scintigraphy. The patient ingests a radiolabeled substance that is accompanied by foods and fluids. The path and rate of movement are followed. Endoscopy or upper gastrointestinal x-rays can also diagnose the disease. **Treatment** is directed at minimizing symptoms and complications. Treatment requires using medications that stimulate contraction of gastric muscles, such as Reglan, Propulsid or Bethanechol. Medications to treat symptoms, such as antacids, may be used. Most importantly, careful control of blood sugar is imperative. **Complications** may include obstruction from bezoars, malnutrition and fluctuations in blood sugar.

Dumping Syndrome

Dumping syndrome results from food entering the small intestines as a rapid rate. This may be due to a surgical complication from stomach surgery or vagotomy. Early **symptoms** include sweating and tachycardia. There may also be abdominal pain and bloating. These symptoms occur between 15 to 30 minutes after the beginning of a meal. Later symptoms resemble hypoglycemia, with sweating, faintness, shakiness and hunger. These symptoms occur between 90 and 120 minutes after the beginning of a meal. **Diagnosis** can be accomplished with endoscopy or barium x-ray studies. **Treatment** may include use of acarbose, which interferes with carbohydrate absorption, for late dumping symptoms. Early dumping may be treated with octreotide, a somatostatin analogue. This reduces certain secretions of hormones.

Small Intestines

Anatomy

The **small intestines** connect the stomach to the large intestines. It is approximately 600 centimeters long and is coiled within the abdominal cavity. It begins at the pyloric sphincter, the outlet of the stomach, and extends to the ileocecal valve, the start of the large intestines.

The small intestines can be divided into **three parts:**

- The *duodenum* is 25 centimeters long and is connected to the stomach at the pyloric sphincter. This is the shortest and widest part of the small intestine and is shaped like a C. It ends at the ligament of Treitz.
- The *jejunum* is 200 centimeters long and connects the duodenum to the ileum.
- The *Ileum* is 300 centimeters long. It extends to the ileocecal valve where the large intestines start. The ileocecal valve controls the flow of contents into the large intestines.

Blood and Nerve Supply

The small intestine is **supplied with blood** from two different contributors.

- The duodenum's needs are met by the *hepatic artery*.
- The balance of the small intestine is supplied from the *superior mesenteric artery*.

Drainage of blood from these organs is accomplished through the superior mesenteric vein. The small intestines are supplied with parasympathetic and sympathetic **nerves** via the enteric plexus. This is composed of the Meissner's plexus in the submucosa, the Auerbach's plexus in the muscular layers and the subserosal contribution. Parasympathetic stimulation increases contraction, secretory function and tone. Sympathetic innervation causes decreased motion and activity. Each villus is supplied by its own blood, lymph and nerve supply.

Cross Sectional Layers

The small intestine has **four layers**.

- The *outermost layer* is composed of serosa and connective tissue.
- The next layer is the *muscularis layer*, composed of an inner layer of circular fibers and outer layer of longitudinal fibers. Between these two muscle bands is the myenteric plexus, a collection of nerves.
- This is followed by the *submucosa layer*, made up of connective tissue, blood vessels, lymphatics and nerves.
- The innermost layer is the *mucosa layer*. The interior part of this is composed of columnar epithelium cells, followed by a band of connective tissue or the lamina propria, and then a layer of smooth muscle.

Mucosal Surface

The **mucosal surface** is structured to provide increased surface area for absorption of nutrients. The plicae circulares, formed by the mucosal and submucosal layers, form folds along the length of the small intestines. The surface is fringed with villi that jut into the *lumen*. Multiple microvilli extend from the surface of each villi. All these projections allow for more area for absorption. The *crypts of Lieberkuhn*, small glands, fall between the villi. These glands generate a new supply of columnar epithelium to replace the mucosal surface regularly. At the base of each of these are *Paneth cells,* which are thought to aid in controlling the microbiologic population in the intestine. *Brunner's glands*, which contain mucous and secretory cells, occur in the duodenum, and these secretions flow into the crypts.

Immune Contributions

The small intestine has abundant **lymphoid tissue**, making up 25% of the mucosal surface. The lymphoid tissue is composed of three different entities:

- Peyer's patches
- Lymphocytes
- Plasma cells

Peyer's patches, which occur in the ileum, are collection of lymphoid tissue. These areas help in antibody production for the body. They participate in the body's immune system. The **lamina propria** contains both lymphocytes and plasma cells, which produce mainly immunoglobin A. This antibody protects the mucosal surface. The **intraepithelial lymphocytes** lurk within the epithelial cells and are largely T cells, which are involved in the immunologic function of the body.

Function

The small intestines **function** to absorb nutrients and to secrete substances to help in processing food. These substances include mucus, digestive aids and various hormones. The small intestine also moves its contents toward the large intestine for continued processing. The secretory function is carried out by a number of different cells. The secretion of substances from the microvilli causes digestion of proteins and carbohydrates. Mucus is secreted by goblet cells around the villi. Other cells contribute mucus, hormones and other substances. The small intestines also receive contributions from the liver and pancreas to aid in digestion. In addition, the Brunner's glands of duodenum protect against the acidity of the stomach chyme.

Absorption Process

The small intestines are responsible for **absorbing the nutritional substances** that are essential to the body. The act of absorption occurs through some basic mechanisms, including hydrolysis, nonionic movement, passive diffusion, facilitated diffusion and active transport. In addition, different substances enter via the small intestine at different sites. Conversely, the same substance can be absorbed by different mechanisms as it passes through the small intestines. In general, the duodenum absorbs Calcium and Iron; the jejunum absorbs fats, proteins and carbohydrate, and the ileum takes in vitamin B12 and bile acids. B12 is absorbed in the distal ileum by an active process employing Intrinsic factor. Water soluble vitamins are usually absorbed by diffusion, however. Potassium is absorbed with sodium in the jejunum, but in the ileum, it is actively absorbed. Calcium is absorbed through several different mechanisms.

Meckel's Diverticulum

In 2% of the population, the ileum has a small congenital anomaly called a **Meckel's diverticulum.** It is an outpouching off of the ileum with a mucosal surface similar to the small intestine. However, this vestigial pouch can also contain gastric and/or pancreatic cells, as well. Release of substances from these aberrant cells can lead to damage and bleeding in adjacent tissue. Meckel's diverticulum is at risk for obstruction from volvulus or intussusception. This can cause pain, vomiting or bleeding. **Diagnosis** requires a radioisotope scan that detects abnormal secretion in the Meckel's diverticulum. Surgery is required to either remove the Meckel's diverticulum or, in some cases, the surrounding small intestinal tissue.

Infections of Small Intestines

The small intestines can be **infected** by organisms that behave in different ways in the bowel. These include:

- Enterotoxigenic bacteria that stimulate secretions in the small bowel causing watery diarrhea, i.e. *Escherichia coli, Vibrio cholerae*
- Bacteria that invade the mucosal surface, causing bloody stools and fever, i.e. *Clostridium difficile, Vibrio cholerae* and *parahaemolyticus*
- Bacteria that invade beneath the mucosal surface, causing systemic illness, i.e. *Yersinia enterocolitica* and *Salmonella typhi*
- Viruses that cause diarrhea, i.e. Norwalk virus and rotavirus.

Diagnosis requires evaluating exposures and travel and evaluation of stools by cultures and stains. Treatment requires fluid replacement and appropriate antibiotics for identified organisms.

Giardiasis

Giardiasis affects the proximal small bowel by the parasite *Giardia lamblia.* The organism gains entry via contaminated water or food. Once ingested, the cysts release trophozoites, which cling to the intestinal lining. Although most are asymptomatic, some exhibit diarrhea. Children may also complain of pain, and headaches, along with nausea and vomiting. **Diagnosis** can be accomplished by evaluating the stool for parasites and Giardia antigen. Endoscopy can also be done to collect specimens of contents and mucosa. Flagyl is the drug of choice. Repeat cultures may be done after treatment. Sometimes a second course is required. If infection persists, patients can be given Atabrine and Flagyl for two weeks.

Cryptosporidiosis and Diphyllobothriasis

In the past, **Cryptosporidiosis** was extremely rare. With the appearance of the AIDS epidemic, with its concomitant immunosuppression, cases have increased in number. The disease is the result of infection by the *Cryptosporidium* parasite by fecal-oral route from animals to humans. It can also be water-borne.

- The disease may last for only a few days to weeks. For the immunocompromised host, however, infection can be fatal.
- The disease is *diagnosed* by checking the stool for the parasite or by evaluating small bowel tissue.
- *Treatment* measures depend on the severity of symptoms. At a minimum, fluid and electrolyte status must be normalized. For those with severe cases, treatment can include Flagyl or other drugs.

Diphyllobothriasis, a fish tapeworm, strikes those who consume raw fish. The tapeworm, which attaches to the intestinal lining, may cause B12 deficiency. Therefore, patients may have no symptoms until the B12 deficiency causes nerve symptoms. *Diagnosis* is accomplished by stool examination. *Treatment* is with Niclosamide.

Infestations by Strongyloidiasis and Ascariasis

Strongyloidiasis is caused by the intestinal parasite, *Strongyloides stercoralis.* Patients develop fever, skin rash and cough, followed by gastrointestinal symptoms. Since the life cycle of this parasite can occur in one person, there is the possibility that the individual can become hyperinfected. The hyperinfected patient has more severe and widespread disease and is at risk for lethal complications. Diagnosis can be accomplished with small intestinal biopsy, X-rays, stool tests and blood tests. Treatment requires the use of thiabendazole.

Ascariasis results from infection by the parasite Ascaris lumbricoides, which is commonly found in the southeastern United States. Once the parasite egg is ingested, it remains in the gut for about 6 months. At that time, it passes through the intestinal wall and enters the circulation, causing fever, coughing and hemoptysis. Patients may complain of pain or change in bowel habits. A common complication is obstruction. Diagnosis is accomplished by stool examination. Treatment requires use of mebendazole. Surgery may be needed to relieve obstruction.

Crohn's Disease

Crohn's disease is one of the diseases classified as inflammatory bowel disease. Although it is more likely to affect the distal ileum, it can involve any part of the gastrointestinal tract. The disease causes inflammation in the submucosal area in a patchy pattern. The actual cause is not known, but some suspected participants are immunologic mechanisms, infections agents or genetics. The disease alternates between inflammatory attacks and relative quiet. When active, the disease causes abdominal pain, nausea, and bloody diarrhea. These symptoms can be severe, and patients can suffer from malnutrition. Children may present with failure to thrive. In some patients, the disease causes extra-intestinal symptoms, such as arthritis, skin lesions and eye inflammation. **Diagnosis** is accomplished with X-rays or endoscopy. Endoscopy offers the advantage of obtaining tissue for diagnosis. **Treatment** is directed at the inflammatory process with drugs such as sulfasalazine, steroids or agents that alter immune responses. **Complications** include obstruction, bleeding, stricture formation, and malabsorption. These complications must be treated accordingly.

Vitamin B12 Deficiency

Vitamin B12 is absorbed in the terminal ileum by the aid of intrinsic factor, which is released by the parietal cell of the stomach lining. It is an essential vitamin, but symptoms of a deficiency take a long time to manifest themselves. A number of different abnormalities lead to this disorder. Some of those include pernicious anemia, loss of gastric mucosal surface, or diseases that disrupt the distal ileum. **Diagnosis** can be made using the Schilling test, a test that measures the path of radio-isotope labeled B12 with and without added intrinsic factor. **Treatment** may require use of B12, but it also includes correcting any underlying abnormalities that interfere with B12 absorption.

Celiac Disease

Celiac disease is a genetic disorder that affects 1 in 300 Americans. These individuals are unable to tolerate gluten, which is found in wheat, barley, rye and possibly oats. Ingesting products containing gluten causes an immunologic reaction in the intestines. The surface of the intestines is damaged, and the villi are flattened. This results in a decreased ability to absorb nutrients. This leads to malabsorption and malnutrition. Although the specific cause is not known, risk factors for the disease include a family history of the disease, being a woman and being of northwestern Europe descent. Symptoms of gluten exposure include abdominal cramping, bloating, gas and diarrhea. If malabsorption develops, other systemic problems may develop, such as osteoporosis from lack of calcium absorption.

Diagnosis and Treatment

Celiac disease is **diagnosed** by a blood antibody test. Additionally, an upper endoscopy with a small bowel biopsy obtains tissue for diagnosis. Sampling of the small bowel should occur in the distal ileum and the jejunum. The tissue has a characteristic flattened appearance, due to the atrophy of the villi. There are many false negatives with biopsy, however, because the entire intestinal wall is not affected simultaneously. Thus, disease can be missed. A positive biopsy, on the other hand, demonstrates that the patient has celiac disease. Some Celiac patients suffer from Dermatitis herpetiformis. Although the specific cause is not known, those individuals develop blistering skin lesions over the elbows and/or knees. Treatment is strict avoidance of any gluten-containing products, which is often not an easy task.

Whipple's Disease and Tropical Sprue

Whipple's disease is quite rare and presents with abdominal pain, diarrhea, arthralgias and malabsorption. The cause is unknown.

- *Diagnosis* is accomplished by obtaining tissue from the small bowel. Examination of the tissue reveals macrophages and cytoplasmic granules.
- *Treatment* requires a 2-week course of intravenous antibiotics. After completion of this course, the patient is given 10-12 months of Tetracycline.

Tropical sprue strikes those in the tropics, causing diarrhea and malabsorption. The intestinal wall undergoes progressive changes, with flattened villi and inflammatory cell collections. Treatment may require using folic acid and tetracycline.

Short Bowel Syndrome

Short bowel syndrome is caused by a decrease in the available length of the small intestine. This can be the result of resection, congenital abnormalities, or Crohn's disease. Since the small intestine is needed for absorption of nutrients, those with short bowel syndrome suffer from malabsorption and malnutrition. The deficiencies in nutrients depend on the area of bowel involved. An important consideration is the ileocecal valve. This is the gatekeeper for food entering the large intestine. It also is a barrier to the encroachment of large intestinal micro flora spreading into the small intestine, which might further exacerbate the problems. These patients need nutritional support. This is usually accomplished with enteral nutrition. The bowel makes certain compensations for the shortened bowel, but the patient needs nourishment to support them, at least in the short term.

Small Bowel Tumors

Tumors of the small bowel include:

- **Primary small intestinal tumors** are not particularly common, accounting for less than 5% of all gastroenteric tumors. These tumors include lymphomas, alpha heavy chain disease, carcinoma, carcinoid tumors or hamartomas.
- The **Peutz-Jeghers syndrome** causes hamartomas in the gastrointestinal tract, usually in the small bowel.
- **Hamartomas** are benign tumors that are composed of normal tissue that is collected in a disorganized mass. Other distinguishing features of this syndrome are pigmentation of the skin.
- **Primary tumors** of the small bowel can occur and are predominantly adenocarcinomas.
- **Secondary tumors** are most likely caused by breast cancer, lung cancer or melanoma.
- **Alpha heavy chain disease** results from the abnormal production of the heavy chain of immunoglobulin A. This leads to malabsorption. This usually progresses to malignant lymphoma.
- **Carcinoid tumors** are more likely to be found in the ileum and appendix.

Carcinoid Syndrome

Carcinoid tumors are often asymptomatic, coming to notice by accident. These tumors can cause problems to patients by causing obstruction. Approximately 1/3 of these tumors are found in the small bowel, and they are often multiple. Some of these can metastasize, particularly to the liver. The syndrome results from the tumor secreting excess hormones that result in various symptoms, such as flushing, wheezing, and diarrhea. A high percentage of patients develop right heart fibrosis, particularly of the tricuspid valve. **Diagnosis** can be done by endoscopic biopsy of tissue or by direct biopsy of the tumor via the abdominal wall. Surgical removal should be attempted if possible. Chemotherapy and radiation have had limited success. Medical treatment should be directed at symptoms.

Large Intestine

Gross Anatomy

The **large intestine** extends from the ileocecal valve to the anus in an upside-down U shape outlining the abdomen. It is 4 to 5 feet long and it is composed of 5 sections: the ascending colon, the transverse colon, the descending colon, the sigmoid colon and the rectum. The large intestine starts at the ileocecal valve, which controls influx from and reflux to the small intestine. This area of the large intestine is called the cecum, which has the appendix affixed to it. Digestive contents move from the cecum to the ascending colon, which runs along the periphery of the right side of the abdomen. At the liver, it bends to run across the top of the abdomen as the transverse colon. At the spleen, located in the upper left quadrant of the abdomen, the colon again bends to head down the left side of the abdomen. At the lower left quadrant of the abdomen, the colon forms an S-shaped contortion, referred to as the sigmoid colon. This then joins the rectum above the pelvic area.

- 31 -

<u>Outer Three Layers in Cross-Section of Intestine Wall</u>

The large intestinal wall is composed of **four layers**:

- The *serosa* covers all of the large intestine but the rectum.
- The *muscularis* is made up of the tenia coli, an inner band of circular muscle and an outer band of longitudinal muscle. Auerbach's plexus, a collection of nerves, is nestled between these layers. Since these are not as long as the intestine itself, the tenia coli compresses the intestinal wall into folds. These small puckers are called haustra.
- Next to this is the *submucosal layer*, composed of connective tissue, blood vessels, lymphatics and nerves, part of which is the Meissner's nerve plexus.
- The *muscularis mucosae*, composed of smooth muscles, separate this layer from the mucosal layer.

<u>Mucosal Surface</u>

The **mucosal surface** is flat and is lined by columnar epithelial cells and goblet cells. The large intestine also has the crypts of Lieberkuhn that line the intestine. The large intestine does not have villi. The inner lining of the large bowel is gathered in folds, referred to as the plicae semilunares. Unlike the rest of the large intestine, the rectum does not have a serosal layer. The mucosal layer is composed of rectal columns, or longitudinal rows, which each have an artery and vein. This mucosal layer meets the anal area at the mucocutaneous border. This border is also where the blood supply and nerve supply changes.

<u>Blood Supply and Innervation</u>

The large intestine is supplied by different **arteries**.

- On the right side, the large intestine is supplied by blood from the superior mesenteric artery.
- On the left side, the large intestine is supplies by the inferior mesenteric artery. Venous blood returns to the circulation via the inferior and superior mesenteric veins.

The balance of the large intestine, the rectum and anal canal, are supplied by a branch of the inferior mesenteric artery, the hemorrhoidal artery. The rectum also is supplied by the hypogastric artery. Venous drainage varies in this area. In the rectum, the blood flows into the superior hemorrhoidal veins, which join the portal veins. The anal area returns its venous blood through the inferior hemorrhoidal veins. Parasympathetic innervation of the large intestine leads to increased activity and secretion; it also inhibits the rectal sphincter. Sympathetic nerves reduce activity and secretions, while stimulating the rectal sphincter.

<u>Function</u>

The motility of the colon operates to mix contents and to help absorb contents. The waste products are eliminated by action of the internal and external sphincter. Movement is slower in the large intestine than in the small intestine. The large intestine more readily absorbs water than does the small intestine. The bulk of this takes place in the ascending colon. The large intestine is populated by normal flora, or organisms. These organisms allow for help in breaking down waste material, breaking down bile acids, production of vitamin K, control of overpopulation by certain undesirable bacteria, and inactivating pancreatic enzymes. These same organisms can be deleterious, as well, by participating in colitis, diarrhea and infections. Passage of material from the rectum is controlled by two sphincters: the internal sphincter and the external sphincter. The internal sphincter, made of smooth muscle, and an external sphincter, made of striated muscle. Voluntary control of the bowels is the function of the levator ani muscles, which surround the rectum.

Diseases that Present with Multiple Polyps

There are several diseases characterized by multiple **polyps**, including juvenile polyps, familial polyposis coli, Gardner's syndrome and Peutz-Jeghers syndrome.

- *Juvenile polyps* occur in young people, usually before the age of 5. This entity is rare after adolescence.
- *Familial polyposis coli* is a disorder that runs in families resulting in multiple polyps. Once the diagnosis is established, surgery to remove the polyps needs to be done. These polyps can become cancerous.
- *Gardner's syndrome* is also a familial disease. Patients develop polyps and osteomas. Since the polyps can become cancerous, surgery is necessary to remove the polyps.
- *Peutz-Jeghers syndrome* causes hamartomas in the large intestines. These individuals also have pigmented lesions on the skin. Although these lesions can become cancerous, many cause no problems.

Angiodysplasia

Angiodysplasia can be found anywhere in the gastrointestinal tract, but these lesions occur most commonly in the cecum and ascending colon. Angiodysplasia refers to a collection of dilated blood vessels, associated with the elderly. Although angiodysplasia is often asymptomatic, it can present with gastrointestinal bleeding. Differentiating this disease from other possible causes of bleeding can be very difficult. **Diagnosis** is accomplished by colonoscopy or angiography. Resection of the affected area clears the problem. Other treatments may include electrocautery or laser. These latter techniques have higher complication rates in this patient population, however.

IBS

Irritable bowel syndrome, or IBS, is marked by motility problems of the intestine without demonstrable organic disease. Patients suffer with alterations of diarrhea and constipation and pain usually in the form of ulcerative colitis and/or Crohn's disease. **Treatment** includes a high-fiber diet, drugs for abdominal pain and psychosocial support. Children present with a recurrent complaint of pain, called chronic recurrent abdominal pain syndrome. They have intermittent bouts without any organic abnormality. Some children also have dizziness, headache and nausea. Drugs are discouraged, but psychological support is emphasized.

Ischemic Colitis

Ischemic colitis is caused by a lack of blood supply to an area of the small or large intestine. This abnormality is more likely to occur at the splenic flexure or in the sigmoid colon. The blood supply to the bowel can be obstructed by embolic events. The blood supply can also be compromised by systemic illnesses that cause hypotension, which leads to a failure to perfuse the bowel. The onset of ischemic colitis is characterized by abrupt pain, fever, abdominal distention, and bloody diarrhea. X-ray findings reveal abnormalities in the mucosa of the affected area in what is called a "thumbprint" pattern. The course of the disease is usually self-limited. Some individuals fail to resolve, going on to develop infarction and peritonitis. These complications require surgical intervention.

Causes of Colitis in Infants

Necrotizing enterocolitis affects neonatal patients. The cause is unclear, but suspected participants include exposure to formula, invasive bacterial infection or some form of ischemic

- 33 -

injury. The disease affects the colon or the distal small intestine, causing bloody stools, distention of the abdomen and vomiting. X-ray of the bowel reveals air in the intestinal wall or portal system, called pneumatosis intestinalis. Supportive therapy may ease the symptoms, but some infants need surgery. **Cow's milk protein-induced enterocolitis affects children** from birth until 6 months. These children are sensitive to milk exposure and can present with different symptoms including vomiting, diarrhea, failure to thrive, bloody stool and irritability. Diagnosis is made by challenging the infant with milk or obtaining tissue to look for inflammation. Affected children should be switched to hypoallergenic formulas.

Ulcerative Colitis

Inflammatory bowel disease of the large intestine can be either ulcerative colitis or Crohn's disease. **Ulcerative colitis**, which does not affect the small intestine, causes ulcerations in the mucosal surface. Scarring can result in shortening and narrowing of the large intestine. The disease often begins in the distal colon and spreads throughout the rest of the large intestine. The inflammatory process is usually uninterrupted. Patients present with bloody diarrhea, anorexia, fever, abdominal tenderness. There can be symptoms outside of the bowel, such as arthritis, liver problems or sclerosing cholangitis. Patients can have periods of quiescent disease interspersed with flares of activity.

Diagnosis, Treatment, and Complications

The diagnosis of **ulcerative colitis** can be made by appropriate X-ray studies and endoscopic evaluation. **Treatment** requires adequate nutrition with avoidance of foods that cause symptoms. Drugs can also minimize symptoms. These include corticosteroids, 5-aminosalicylate drugs and immunosuppressives. For unresponsive patients, surgery may be needed. **Complications** include toxic megacolon, a distention of the colon, which requires immediate intervention. This complication can lead to perforation, infection or bleeding. At first, the patient may respond to antibiotics, bowel rest and fluid support. Surgery may be necessary to remove the colon. Patients with ulcerative colitis are at increased risk of colon cancer and need to be followed carefully.

Pseudomembranous Colitis

Pseudomembranous colitis involves inflammation of the mucosal layer with areas covered by a pseudomembrane. This disease is usually associated with an exposure to a toxin, such as an antibiotic. Patients develop diarrhea, crampy pain and fever. Most cases are the result of an overgrowth of the organism, *Clostridium difficile*. There have been cases of pseudomembranous colitis caused by other organisms, but this is rare. **Diagnosis** is accomplished by endoscopy and biopsy. Stools can also be evaluated for the presence of the toxin. **Treatment** requires a course of antibiotics and possibly administering medications that bind the organism. Although most people have resolution of symptoms, some need to be hospitalized.

Crohn's Disease of the Large Intestine

Crohn's disease, another form of inflammatory bowel disease, can affect the small or large intestine. The inflammatory process involves the entire thickness of the gut wall and is not necessarily continuous. *The symptoms are similar to ulcerative colitis, but pain is more pronounced.* Like ulcerative colitis, Crohn's disease may affect areas outside the bowel, such as joints, the skin and the liver. **Treatment** is aimed at quelling the inflammation. Fluid and electrolyte support help maintain the patient's status. Drugs can offer some anti-inflammatory aid. Some drugs include the 5-aminosaliclate drugs, corticosteroids, and immunosuppressive drugs. **Complications** include bleeding, stricture formation, fistula formation and perforation.

- 34 -

Radiation Enteritis

Radiation enteritis results from injury to the abdomen from radiation therapy. If the bowel wall is affected, patients develop a change in bowel habits, diarrhea and tenesmus. Those affected during treatment develop an acute form of the disease. Patients present with nausea, cramps and changes in routine bowel movements. If chronic damage develops, patients develop bleeding, strictures, obstruction and perforation. These symptoms may develop anywhere from 3 months to 30 years after radiation treatment. The chronic form of this disease can be progressive and resistant to treatment. Use of intralumenal steroids or sulfasalazine may help. Surgery may be needed for those with serious abnormalities, such as obstruction or perforation.

Parasitic Diseases of the Colon

Amebiasis is caused by the parasite *Entamoeba histolytica*. Infection is most often by fecal-oral contamination. Symptoms may include diarrhea, appendicitis or abscesses in organs. Some individuals develop dysentery, with fever, nausea and vomiting. Stool evaluation reveals the parasite. Other possible ways to diagnosis amebiasis include sigmoidoscopy or barium enema. Abscesses are diagnosed via X-rays or biopsies. Treatment requires Yodoxin, often accompanied by Flagyl.

Trypanosomiasis is a parasitic disease, called Chagas' disease, caused by *Trypanosoma cruzi*. It is transmitted by a bug bite, along with several other methods. The organism causes an intense inflammation locally and may become blood borne. It tends to invade the heart, the esophagus and the colon, destroying nervous tissue. This leads to enlargement of the affected organ. Diagnosis is made by finding the parasite in the blood or tissue. Extended use of the drug Lampit is needed to treat the disease.

Trichuriasis, or whipworm, is caused by *Trichuris trichiura*. The parasite is spread by fecal-oral contamination, congregating in the cecum and ascending colon. Diagnosis is made by stool examination, and the infection responds well to mebendazole (Vermox).

Diverticulosis and Diverticulitis

Diverticulitis is an infection of a diverticulum. Diverticula are bulging sacs formed in the colon. These protrusions, evidence of **diverticulosis**, are formed at weakened areas of the intestinal wall, and are prone to infection, called **diverticulitis**. These abnormalities can occur anywhere in the colon, but are more commonly found in the descending and sigmoid colon located in the left side of the abdominal cavity. The occurrence of diverticula increases with age, and rarely occurs in those younger than 40. Other potential contributing factors may include lack of dietary fiber, constipation, and obesity. Although most patients with diverticulosis have no symptoms, a few present with complaints, such as constipation, cramps, diarrhea or bloating. The patient with diverticulitis displays abdominal pain, constipation, and fever.

Treatment and Complications

Treatment includes appropriate antibiotics and a low-fiber, liquid diet. If diverticulitis does not respond to treatment or recurs frequently, surgery may need to be performed. The affected area, usually located in the sigmoid colon, is drained and the section with the diverticulum is removed. **Complications** of diverticulitis include abscess formation, obstruction and peritonitis. An abscess, or collection of pus, can form. Infrequently, the infection can spread into the abdominal cavity, causing peritonitis. This is a grave complication. Intestinal obstruction can occur, as well. Because of the swelling or possible scarring from the infected diverticula, the ability to move intestinal contents can be blocked. The obstruction needs to be treated to avoid intestinal perforation.

Colon Cancer

Colon cancer is one of the most common forms of cancer in this country. If detected early, the prognosis is good. Because of that, the American Cancer Society recommends screening the population for colon cancer. Depending on age and risk, the recommendations may include sigmoidoscopy, colonoscopy or stool evaluation for blood. Those at increased risk include patients with a family history of colon cancer, people with high risk diseases, like ulcerative colitis or familial polyposis, or a prior history of certain cancers. The majority of tumors are **adenocarcinomas,** which are usually located in the cecum, ascending colon or sigmoid colon. Tumors of the right side of the bowel have the onset of symptoms later in the disease process, but can include blood in the stool, weight loss, anorexia and pain. Surgery may be used for treatment or for palliation. Patients may also receive radiation, chemotherapy or both.

Intestinal Obstruction

The large intestine can be **obstructed** by many different entities, such as cancers, strictures, or polyps. Impingement on the lumen can also occur from extra-intestinal causes, such as visceral tumors. The causes of the obstruction can be categorized into three main groups:

- Mechanical
- Neurogenic
- Vascular

Patients present with pain, nausea, vomiting and distention. An obstruction can present with different effects. If the blood supply is not affected, the obstruction is called simple. If the blood supply is impinged upon, the obstruction is called strangulated. If the blood supply is totally interrupted, it is called incarcerated. **Diagnosis** may be accomplished by careful evaluation and X-ray studies.

One form of **mechanical obstruction** of the large intestine is Hirschsprung's disease, a congenital lack of neuronal tissue. The lack of this innervation inhibits the bowel's ability to relax, causing the dilation of the bowel. *Symptoms* may include diarrhea, nausea, vomiting, constipation, or perforation. The most dreaded complication is ischemia from overdistention. *Diagnosis* is made by Barium enema and tissue biopsy. *Treatment* requires surgery to remove the effected colon segments. Intestinal pseudo-obstruction, a form of **neurogenic obstruction,** results from poor intestinal motility. Patients present with weight loss and intermittent abdominal distention. An X-ray picture of paralytic ileus is seen, with fluid levels in dilated bowel. There is a chronic form of this disorder that may be associated with other organic diseases. **Vascular obstruction** results when the blood supply to the intestine is interrupted by embolic disease or atherosclerotic disease. The resulting ischemia can lead to a life-threatening illness.

Biliary System

The gallbladder and its associated ducts comprise the **biliary system.** The gallbladder stores bile that is made by the liver. Bile, a greenish-yellowish fluid, functions to eliminate wastes from the liver and to help break down fat during digestions. When food is ingested, the gallbladder is stimulated to contract by the enzyme cholecystokinin-pancreozymin. This contraction forces the bile into the cystic duct, which joins with the hepatic duct to form the common bile duct. The common bile duct passes through the head of the pancreas and joins the pancreatic duct. Bile, along with pancreatic enzymes, flows into the duodenum through the ampulla of Vater. This opening into the duodenum is controlled by a muscular structure, the sphincter of Oddi. It regulates the flow of bile and pancreatic secretions into the small bowel and restricts reflux from the intestinal tract.

<u>Composition of Bile</u>

Bile is composed largely water. Most of the water is re-absorbed, however. It also consists of bile salts, fatty acids, lipids, bilirubin, and other substances.

- Bile functions to provide a means of eliminating waste products from the liver.
- It is also a key factor in digesting and absorbing certain nutrients and activating certain digestive enzymes.
- It also functions to counteract the acidic content in the duodenum and to facilitate the absorption of some minerals. When the flow of bile is obstructed, the concentration of bile in the blood increases. The excess bilirubin is deposited in various tissues, like the sclera of the eye, giving that tissue a yellowish hue or jaundice.

Cholelithiasis

Cholelithiasis or gallstones are formed when abnormal concentrations of cholesterol, bile or bilirubin harden into a stone. A slow-emptying gallbladder can increase the chance of forming stones. Gallstones are usually composed of cholesterol or a mixture including cholesterol. About 20% are pigmented stones, composed of bilirubin mixed with other substances. They can be tiny or the size of a golf ball. Patients may have one stone or many. The risk of forming concretions depends on the makeup of the stones. Cholesterol stones are increased in females, with exposure to estrogen, with some hyperlipidemias, and with certain drugs. Pigmented stones are more likely to occur in those with hemolysis, alcoholism, total parenteral nutrition, and biliary infections.

<u>Symptoms and Treatment</u>

Often **gallstones** are asymptomatic, but they can cause symptoms when they increase in size or if they cause obstruction. If a patient develops symptoms, these symptoms commonly follow a fatty meal or occur at night. *Symptoms* include pain, nausea, vomiting, indigestion, jaundice, fever, chills. **Diagnosis** is made by abdominal ultrasound. Also X-ray studies can be done. If these are negative, but the symptoms are suggestive of biliary disease, an ERCP may be done. **Treatment** for symptomatic stones usually involves surgery to remove the gallbladder or cholecystectomy. With symptomatic pigmented stones, surgery is the only option. The treatment for cholesterol stones, on the other hand, has some alternative choices. Certain medications can potentially dissolve these stones. In addition, biliary lithotripsy can be used. This involves using sound waves through the abdominal wall to dissolve the stones.

Cholecystitis

Cholecystitis is inflammation of the gallbladder. Although this can occur without gallstones, this is rare except in the pediatric population. It is most commonly due to an obstruction of the cystic duct by a gallstone, or acute calculous cholecystitis. Risk factors may include obesity, diabetes, hemolytic anemia or pregnancy. Symptoms may include abdominal pain, fever, nausea, vomiting, and pain exacerbation when consuming fatty foods. **Diagnosis** may be accomplished with ultrasound or radioisotope imaging studies. Although removing the gallbladder is the best treatment, not every patient can undergo the procedure. With those patients, a cholecystostomy may be done, providing drainage via a temporary tube placement. This can be accomplished by ERCP, by surgery or by percutaneous drainage. **Complications** may include perforation, peritonitis, or gallstone ileus.

Primary Sclerosing Cholangitis

Primary sclerosing cholangitis is a disease that causes strictures in the bile ducts. The obstruction to the flow of bile can lead to liver disease. The majority of patients have a history of ulcerative colitis; it can also be seen with Crohn's disease. This disease affects men more commonly than women and can occur in relatively young patients. Individuals with this disease may develop jaundice, pruritis, pain and liver dysfunction. Diagnosis is accomplished by ERCP, ultrasonography or biopsy. Treatment for advanced disease requires liver transplant. Without a transplant, symptomatic patients go on to develop liver failure and portal hypertension. There is an increased risk for the development of cholangiosarcoma in these patients.

Cancers of the Biliary System

Gallbladder cancer is most often adenocarcinomas. These cancers spread locally or lymphatic metastasis. Patients complain of pain, anorexia, and weight loss. These tumors often co-exist with gallstones. **Diagnosis** may be accomplished by imaging studies, such as cholangiograms, or by ERCP. **Treatment** is directed at symptomatic relief. Surgery may be performed for small tumors, but invasive therapy has little benefit. For symptoms of obstruction, a stent may be placed to relieve the obstruction and reduce the risk of infection. The prognosis is poor, with a five-year survival rate of 5%. The most common form of cancer in the biliary system is adenocarcinoma. Patients present with jaundice, intermittent abdominal pain, nausea and weight loss. At diagnosis, the cancer is usually found to have spread. Although surgery can be done to remove the tumor, the prognosis is poor. Children are at risk of developing botryoid embryonal rhabdomyosarcoma, a tumor with a poor prognosis.

Pancreas

Anatomy

The **pancreas** stretches across the upper abdomen, starting behind the duodenum and stomach and ending behind the spleen. The pancreas functions as both an exocrine and an endocrine organ. The exocrine cells, or acinar cells, are cuboidal cells that cluster around a network of ducts. These ducts connect to the duct of Wirsung, which travels through the entire organ, collecting secretions. This central duct meets the common bile duct and these two systems drain into the duodenum. The endocrine function of the pancreas is carried out by the endocrine cells located in the islets of Langerhans. These cells comprise about 1% of the pancreatic cells.

Endocrine and Exocrine Function

The **endocrine function** of the pancreas is performed by three different endocrine cells that secrete their products directly into the blood.

- The *alpha cells* release glucagon when there is a drop in blood sugar concentration. This substance increases glucose in the blood by promoting glucose formation from glycogen stored in the liver.
- The *beta cells* are stimulated to release insulin when the blood sugar level is high, allowing cells to act on glucose through metabolism or storage.
- The exocrine function of the pancreas is due to the secretion of pancreatic enzymes by *acinar cells*. The main enzymes include amylases for carbohydrate absorption, lipases for fat digestion and proteases for protein digestion.

- 38 -

Acute Pancreatitis

Acute pancreatitis is the abrupt onset of an inflammation of the pancreas. There are many causes, including gallstone obstruction, alcohol, infections, drugs, hyperlipidemias and hyperparathyroidism. *Symptoms* include pain, nausea, vomiting, fever and possibly shock. Blood tests reveal an elevated amylase and lipase. Further details are obtained by imaging studies, ultrasound or endoscopic studies. **Treatment** is supportive, sometimes requiring intensive care. Depending on the cause, different therapies may be offered, such as antibiotics. If gallstones are the cause of the pancreatitis, the patient will need surgery or ERCP. **Necrotizing pancreatitis** is a destructive acute pancreatitis that can be very serious. Pancreatic tissue is necrosed and at risk for infection, pseudocyst formation and pancreatic failure. 1/3 of patients die from this form of pancreatitis. **Interstitial pancreatitis** is a milder form that affects interstitial tissue, causing less damage. Some of these cases, however, may require intensive care, as well.

Chronic Pancreatitis

Chronic pancreatitis is the result of continued inflammation, leading to destruction of pancreatic tissue. In this country, alcohol is the most common cause of chronic pancreatitis. Other etiologies to be considered are cystic fibrosis, malnutrition, and familial pancreatitis. *Symptoms* include pain, weight loss, diabetes, and malabsorption. Diagnosis depends on the history, appropriate X-ray studies, and studies involving the cause of the symptoms. **Treatment** is directed at pain relief and control of symptoms. Depending on the cause of the disease, interventions might include ERCP with interventions or surgery. Surgery may be performed to remove parts of the pancreas or to drain areas.

Pancreatic Pseudocysts

Pancreatic pseudocysts are collections of pancreatic materials that are encapsulated without a true epithelial layer. These are associated with both acute and chronic pancreatitis and can be single or multiple. The majority of pseudocysts disappear without intervention. *Symptoms* may include pain, nausea, vomiting, and weight loss. Diagnosis is by imaging studies. If the pseudocyst and its associated symptoms that persist, the pseudocyst may need to be drained. This can be done via surgery, percutaneously or ERCP. Intervention must be provided immediately if the pseudocyst becomes infected, ruptures or hemorrhages. Complications include peritonitis, bleeding and obstruction.

Pancreatic Adenocarcinomas and Cystic Tumors

Pancreatic cancers are mostly adenocarcinomas. Patients complain of pain, vomiting, weakness, and weight loss. *Often patients will develop jaundice.* Diagnosis is accomplished by imaging studies and tissue biopsy, either percutaneously or via ERCP. The prognosis of this disease is poor. Most interventions are for palliation. Surgery, such as the Whipple operation, can be done. Stent placements help with obstructive complications of the biliary tree, duodenum or the pancreas. Pancreatic cystic tumors can occur anywhere in the pancreas, although most often in the head of the pancreas. These tumors contain fluid and are difficult to differentiate from pseudocysts.

Endocrine Tumors

The following are other endocrine tumors of the pancreas:

- **Insulinomas** are beta cell tumors causing hypoglycemia. Usually there is only one tumor.
- **Glucagonomas** are alpha cell tumors causing excess glucagon release. Patients manifest the skin disease, necrolytic migratory erythema, which presents as an erythematous rash that blisters and often develops a bronze pigment in healing. These patients often have concomitant diabetes.
- **Somatostatinomas** have excess somatostatin action, resulting in inhibition of other hormones and enzymes. These patients present with steatorrhea, diabetes and gall stones.
- **Vasoactive intestinal peptide tumors** or Vipomas develop diarrhea, low potassium and low acid output.

Treatment includes surgical removal of the tumors and use of several anti-tumor agents. Streptozocin decreases tumor mass. Other types of tumors may be controlled by a somatostatin analogue.

Exocrine Dysfunction

Pancreatic exocrine insufficiency is due to the reduction in available pancreatic enzymes to aid in digestion. The patient suffers from diarrhea, malabsorption and malnutrition. These individuals need enzyme replacement and nutritional supplements. **Cystic fibrosis** is a hereditary disease that disturbs the exocrine function of the pancreas, as well as the functioning of the respiratory system, the sweat glands and the reproductive system. Mucus production is altered, leading to thickened secretions of mucus. These children suffer from pancreatic insufficiency, respiratory disease and other abnormalities. Testing for electrolytes in the sweat of these individuals shows increased sodium and chloride; DNA can also be tested.

Liver

Anatomy
The **liver,** located in the right upper quadrant of the abdomen, is divided into a large right lobe and a smaller left lobe. Each lobe is further divided into hepatic lobules, composed of six hepatic cells. Each of the lobules is accompanied by the portal triad, consisting of a vein, an artery and a bile duct. Interspersed between these cells are sinusoids lined with Kupffer cells. The Kupffer cells are responsible for removing substances from the blood, such as old red blood cells or debris. Blood is supplied through the portal vein and the portal artery. Blood is drained through the hepatic veins.

Function in Digesting Fat
The **liver functions** to form bile and to participate in metabolism, coagulation, detoxification and storage of vitamins. Bile is used to aid in the digestion of fats. It is composed of bile acids, bile pigments, bilirubin and other substances. Bile acids, which are formed from cholesterol, become bile salts in the liver. Bile pigments are a breakdown product of red blood cells. Bilirubin, one of the bile pigments is released into the blood. Bilirubin, when joined or conjugated with glucuronic acid is excreted in bile. The bile drains into the hepatic ducts and joins the biliary duct system to deliver its contents to the small intestine.

<u>Other Functions</u>

Additional functions of the liver include:

- The liver aids in carbohydrate and protein metabolism.
- It stores, releases and synthesizes glucose, depending on the needs of the body.
- It also metabolizes amino acids, synthesizes protein, metabolizes certain hormones and processes digested fat.
- The liver synthesizes the essential factors for both clotting and anticoagulating the blood.
- The liver cells accomplish detoxification by making toxins more water soluble so they can be disposed of by the body more easily.
- The liver is a reservoir for a number of vitamins, including riboflavin, vitamin D, vitamin K and vitamin E.

Cirrhosis

Cirrhosis of the liver results from the liver's attempts to repair and regenerate after an injury. The resulting inflammation, scarring and anatomical rearrangement leads to liver impairment. One of the major causes of cirrhosis is related to alcohol. The pathology is related to an enlarged liver with fatty infiltrates. Another form of cirrhosis results from bile duct injuries, such as primary biliary cirrhosis. The disease is related to cholestasis, causing fibrosis, inflammation and cell death. **Postnecrotic cirrhosis** follows a severe injury to the liver from infections, hepatotoxins or metabolic diseases. Symptoms may include pain, anorexia, jaundice or bruising. Diagnosis is established by tissue specimen. Those with cirrhosis may develop portal hypertension leading to varices, hepatic encephalopathy, hepatorenal syndrome or ascites. These individuals are also at risk of developing liver cancer.

Complications of Cirrhosis

The hepatorenal syndrome results in kidney failure in individuals with liver disease without evidence of other organic disease involving the kidney. There is gradual renal failure, with decreasing urine output, electrolyte abnormalities, and mental impairment. The prognosis is grim. **Hepatic encephalopathy** results in mental dysfunction in patients with liver disease. This can progress to coma. The cause is uncertain, but may be related to ammonia accumulation. Controlling gastrointestinal bleeding is important, since blood in the gut may increase ammonia levels. Lactulose may be given to bind ammonia in the gut and reducing its absorption.

Portal Hypertension

Portal hypertension is caused when the portal circulation encounters resistance, as in cirrhosis. This results in the shunting of blood through other systems. The excess pressure placed on other circulatory elements results in esophageal and gastric varices, splenomegaly, and hemorrhoids. To ascertain elevated pressures in the portal circulation, measurements must be taken to document a pressure gradient in the portal vein. To relieve the pressure, procedures are instituted to shunt blood away from the areas under pressure. These interventions include: portacaval shunts, splenorenal shunts, mesocaval shunts and TIPS or transjugular intrahepatic portosystemic shunts.

Hepatitis A and B

Hepatitis A is a viral disease that is spread by fecal-oral contamination. Although often asymptomatic, patients can present with fever, jaundice, nausea, pain and an enlarged liver. Most have no complications, but some develop cholestatic jaundice. There is a vaccine available for use.

Those exposed should be given immune globulin. **Hepatitis B** is spread via blood, semen or saliva. Patients develop a non-specific illness, followed by jaundice. Patients develop pain, nausea, fever, jaundice and enlarged livers. Complications may include chronic hepatitis, cirrhosis and liver failure. There is a vaccine available. Interferon can be used to reduce inflammation and aid in clearance of the virus.

Hepatitis C, D, and E

Hepatitis C is a blood borne virus that causes chronic disease in roughly 90% of those infected. 20% of patients develop cirrhosis. Some develop cryoglobulinemia, which is associated with kidney disease and a lower leg rash. Treatment requires the use of interferon, which inhibits viral replication and aids in clearing the virus from liver cells. **Hepatitis D** is a virus only infects individuals with hepatitis B. HDV occurs as a co-infection with hepatitis B, and is eliminated with the hepatitis B infection. As a superinfection, however, HDV increases the severity of hepatitis B. Interferon has been used. **Hepatitis E** is spread by the fecal-oral route. It is prevalent in poorer regions and causes acute disease.

Alcoholic Hepatitis, Drug-Induced Hepatitis, and Non-Alcoholic Steatohepatitis

Alcoholic hepatitis is inflammation related to the ingestion of alcohol. Patients present with abdominal pain, fever, vomiting, enlarged liver and anorexia. This appears to be a precursor of cirrhosis. **Drug-induced hepatitis** is inflammation related to a drug exposure. This reaction can be dose-dependent, idiosyncratic or cholestatic. Some patients may have no symptoms, others may become very sick. Tylenol overdoses can cause fulminant hepatic failure and require treatment with N-acetylcysteine. **Non-alcoholic steatohepatitis** is inflammation of the liver related to increased fatty deposits. It may be related to weight and diabetes. It can progress to cirrhosis.

Liver Cancer

Liver cancer can involve the liver cells or the bile duct cells. Those with an increased risk of developing liver cancer have cirrhosis, hepatitis B or C, and exposure to certain toxins. It commonly spreads to the lungs and peritoneum. Metastatic disease is common in the liver, originating from lung, breast, or gastrointestinal sites. Most patients present with advanced disease, complaining of pain and weight loss. Diagnosis is accomplished by scanning and biopsy. Alpha fetoprotein may also be elevated. For those with limited disease, removal of the tumor may be used. Chemotherapy may treat pain; obstruction may need to be treated with stent placement.

Wilson's Disease and Hemochromatosis

Wilson's disease is a hereditary disease that results in copper build up in the liver, as well as other organs such as the brain or kidney. In the organs with copper deposits, the tissue is destroyed, causing organ failure. A characteristic Kayser-Fleischer ring may be detected as a brown ring around the eye. Treatment requires use of D-penicillamine. All family members need to be evaluated for the presence of the disease. **Hemochromatosis** is a hereditary disease in which iron accumulates in tissues such as the liver, joints, heart and skin. Patients complain of abdominal pain, joint pain, weakness, and skin discoloration. These patients are at an increased risk of hepatocellular carcinoma. Treatment requires phlebotomy to remove iron from the body.

Porphyria Diseases

Porphyria leads to an excess of porphyrins or related substances because of a defect in heme synthesis. The hepatic porphyrias include acute intermittent porphyria, hereditary coproporphyria, variegate porphyria, and porphyria cutanea tarda or PCT. PCT is somewhat different in that there are no abdominal or neurologic symptoms. Instead, patients develop skin lesions, excess hair and some hepatic abnormalities. This disease can be either inherited or acquired. The other listed diseases may present with abdominal pain and neurologic symptoms. Another porphyria disease is **protoporphyria**. Patients are sensitive to light and may have liver disease. Cholestyramine may control the liver disease.

Gastrointestinal Bleeding

Gastrointestinal bleeding can occur anywhere along the gastrointestinal tract. It can be minimal and intermittent to life-threatening hemorrhage. **Some causes of gastrointestinal causes include:**

- Peptic ulcer disease is the most common cause of gastrointestinal bleeding. This refers to an ulcer in the stomach or duodenum.
- Esophageal Varices are a widening of the blood vessels in the lower part of the esophagus and sometimes in the upper part of the stomach.
- Mallory-Weiss tears are lacerations in the esophageal mucosa from vomiting.
- Vascular malformations are abnormal collections of blood vessels that are prone to bleeding.
- Meckel's diverticulum is a vestige of fetal tissue in the small intestine.
- Diverticulosis results in outpouchings of the large intestine that disrupts a blood vessel.
- Angiodysplasia refers to stretched and distorted vessels in the large intestine resulting from aging.
- Hemorrhoids are swollen veins in the lower part of the rectum or anus.
- Neoplasia can occur anywhere along the tract and cause bleeding.
- Esophagitis/Gastritis/Colitis is inflammation of the bowel mucosa.
- Intussusception is the telescoping of one section of intestine into another.
- Obstruction causes complete blockage of the bowel.
- Cancer anywhere in the gastrointestinal tract can cause bleeding.

Patient Education and Advocacy

Pre- and Post- Procedure Patient Education for GI Procedures and Colonoscopy and Esophagogastroduodenoscopy

Patient education in preparation for GI procedures is similar, regardless of the procedure: The patient should clearly understand the name and purpose of the procedure, the risks and benefits, any food restrictions (red meat, red dye) and medication restrictions (such as blood thinners and iron preparations), the GI prep required, the need to be NPO for 6 to 8 hours prior to the procedure, the need to arrange for transportation because of post-sedation grogginess, the type of sedation the patient will receive, the need for an IV during the procedure, and possible complications or adverse reactions. Post-procedure education may vary, depending on the risks associated with the procedure.

Colonoscopy

Patient can resume normal diet. Patient must immediately notify MD for abdominal distention, severe abdominal pain, increased fever, vomiting and rectal bleeding (>30 mL).

- 43 -

Esophagogastroduodenoscopy

Food and drink restricted until swallowing reflex intact. Sore throat may persist for a few days. Patient must immediately notify MD for increased fever, chills, tarry or blood stools, dysphagia, increasing throat pain, chest pain, abdominal distention and pain.

Post-Procedure Education for Endoscopic Retrograde Cholangiopancreatography and Percutaneous Endoscopic Gastrostomy

Endoscopic Retrograde Cholangiopancreatography

Food and drink restricted until swallowing reflex intact. Sore throat may persist for a few days. Patient must immediately notify MD for increased fever, chills, tarry or blood stools, dysphagia, increasing throat pain, chest pain, abdominal distention and pain. Patient should be advised of risk of pancreatitis.

Percutaneous Endoscopic Gastrostomy

Patient must meet with a dietician and have a clear understanding of feeding procedures and adequate nutrition. Patient/Family must learn wound care, skin care, and should notify the MD immediately for signs of infection (redness, swelling, pain) or displacement of the tube. The patient/family must learn how to care for the PEG tube and should practice carrying out feedings under supervision.

Indications and Recommendations for Colonoscopy

Colonoscopy, examination of the colon with a flexible four-foot colonoscope with a light source and video camera at its tip, is indicated for:

- Periodic routine screening for colorectal cancer and colorectal polyps at age 45 to 50 and every 10 years until age 75. Between ages 76 and 85, screening recommendations depend on general condition or risk factors. Screening is not recommended for those over age 85.
- History of colorectal cancer or polyps. Frequency usually increased to every 3 years if precancerous polyps removed.
- History of blood in the stool, which may indicate colon cancer.
- History of change in bowel habits, such as constipation or diarrhea, abdominal pain.
- History of acute/chronic iron-deficiency anemia, which may be related to blood loss.
- History of ulcerative colitis or Crohn's disease, which increases risk of colon cancer.
- History of family genetic conditions associated with colon cancer, such as hereditary nonpolyposis colorectal cancer.

Preventative Measures for Colon Cancer

Preventative measures for colon cancer include:

- Have regular screenings for colon cancer every year with home stool tests, flexible sigmoidoscopy every 5 years, and colonoscopy every 10 years, starting at age 45 or earlier and more frequent if risk factors present (Crohn's disease, family history of colorectal cancer, hereditary conditions, type 2 diabetes, ulcerative colitis, alcoholism).
- Avoid obesity and maintain weight within normal range.
- Stop smoking or don't start.
- Remain physically active, ideally for at least 30 minutes daily.
- Avoid red meat and processed meats, limit to 3 servings or fewer per week.

- Eat a diet with ample fruits, vegetables, and whole grains.
- Avoid simple carbohydrates (sugar, flour).
- Ensure adequate vitamins and minerals, especially vitamin D and calcium.
- Limit intake of alcohol to one drink daily for females and 2 drinks daily for males.

Effects of Substance Use on Gastrointestinal Health

Substance abuse can have profound negative effects on the gastrointestinal system:

- *Alcohol*: Increases acidity in the stomach, leading to stomach ulcers and GI bleeding. Liver becomes scarred, and cirrhosis develops because of the need to metabolize large amounts of alcohol.
- *Opiates/Opioids*: Chronic constipation caused by the drugs may lead to narcotic bowel syndrome with chronic abdominal distention, nausea, vomiting, and constipation. Drugs that include acetaminophen can result in liver damage and lead to liver failure.
- *Tobacco*: Increases the risk of development of peptic ulcers and Crohn's disease. Also increases risk of cancer.
- *Cocaine*: Blood clots associated with use may cause intestinal necrosis. Also increases risks of intestinal and gastric perforations and ulcerations as well as liver damage
- *Methamphetamine*: Tooth decay, loss of teeth, and impaired blood flow to the gums results in "meth mouth" and impaired ability to chew. Constipation or diarrhea are common. The liver and pancreas functions may become impaired, affecting digestion. Absorption of nutrients is impaired. Intestinal infarction may occur.

Patient Advocacy

Patient advocacy in gastroenterology includes:

- Working for the best interests of the patient when an ethical issue arises, despite personal values that might be in conflict.
- Educating patients about their rights and responsibilities.
- Incorporating patients' values into the plan of care.
- Assisting patients and families with resources to make difficult or complex decisions.
- Empowering patients to make decisions.
- Reporting abusive or negligent care and ensuring patient safety.
- Sharing patients' concerns with physicians and other health providers.
- Collaborating with patients in the development of the plan of care.
- Showing respect for the patients and their families.
- Supporting cultural preferences and beliefs.
- Ensuring that patients have adequate knowledge to provide informed consent.
- Engaging in research to promote evidence-based practice.
- Lobbying for improved quality of patient care at the local, state, and national levels.
- Providing follow-up care.
- Promoting routine screening, such as for colon cancer.

Important Terms

Term	Definition
Esophagus	The **esophagus** is a muscular tube that connects the mouth to the stomach.
UES	**UES** or the **upper esophageal sphincter** is the upper end of the esophagus.
LES	**LES** or the **lower esophageal sphincter** is where the esophagus joins the stomach.
Peristalsis	**Peristalsis** describes the rhythmic, coordinated muscular contractions of the gastrointestinal tract.
Dysphagia	**Dysphagia** is the symptom of difficulty swallowing.
Odynophagia	**Odynophagia** is the symptoms of painful swallowing.
Esophageal Varices	**Esophageal varices** are dilated, distended vessels in the esophageal wall.
Zenker's Diverticulum	**Zenker's diverticulum** is an esophageal diverticulum or outpouching that is caused by UES dysfunction.
Esophagitis	**Esophagitis** is an inflammation of the mucosal lining
Mallory-Weiss Tear	**Mallory-Weiss tear** is a laceration in the esophageal lining.
Achalasia	**Achalasia** is a dilation of the esophagus from abnormal peristalsis and/or high LES pressure.
Diffuse Esophageal Spasm	**Diffuse esophageal spasm** is chaotic, simultaneous contractures of the esophageal musculature.
Barrett's Esophagus	**Barrett's esophagus** occurs with the replacement of normal squamous epithelial cells by non-squamous cells in the esophagus.
Nutcracker Esophagus	**Nutcracker esophagus** results from an increase in the amplitude of peristaltic contractions.
Chyme	**Chyme** is a combination of food with stomach secretions.
Dyspepsia	**Dyspepsia** is non-specific epigastric pain or nausea.
Helicobacter pylori	*Helicobacter pylori* are gram negative organisms associated with peptic ulcer disease.
Linitis plastica	**Linitis plastica** is called leather bottle stomach, a diffuse submucosal stomach cancer that causes fibrosis.
Pernicious anemia	**Pernicious anemia** is a vitamin B12 deficiency due to lack of intrinsic factor.
Gastric polyp	**Gastric polyp** is an uncommon stomach lesion that protrudes into the stomach.
Stress ulcers	**Stress ulcers** are gastric ulcers associated with severe stresses, such as illnesses and burns.
Hypertrophic pyloric stenosis	**Hypertrophic pyloric stenosis** occurs in infants and is more common in males. The pyloric sphincter resists passage of food to the intestines. This usually requires surgery.
Rugae	**Rugae** are wrinkles in the stomach surface to allow for expansion.
Parietal cells	**Parietal cells** are responsible for releasing intrinsic factor for vitamin B12 absorption.
Plicae circulares	**Plicae circulares** are the arrangement of the mucosa and submucosa that provides increased surface area in the small intestines.

Term	Definition
Volvulus	**Volvulus** occurs when the bowel twists around itself. It can cause ischemia.
Intussusception	**Intussusception** occurs when part of the intestine telescopes up the lumen of the adjacent intestine.
Borborygmi	**Borborygmi** refers to excessively loud bowel sounds.
Lactase deficiency	**Lactase deficiency** occurs when the small intestinal lining lacks the enzyme lactase, causing diarrhea and malabsorption with lactose products.
Abetalipoproteinemia	**Abetalipoproteinemia** occurs in individuals that lack beta-lipoproteins, which leads to build up of fat in the small intestines. This causes malabsorption.
Intrinsic Factor	**Intrinsic factor** is produced by the gastric parietal cell and allows for absorption of vitamin B12.
Crypts of Lieberkuhn	**Crypts of Lieberkuhn** are the area adjacent to the small intestinal villi responsible for replenishing the columnar epithelium.
Peyer's Patches	**Peyer's patches** are lymph collection/nodes in the ileum.
Steatorrhea	**Steatorrhea** is bulky, malodorous stool with excess fat content.
Hemorrhoids	**Hemorrhoids** are swollen blood vessels in the anal area. Internal hemorrhoids occur above the internal sphincter; external hemorrhoids below. Those from the internal area drain into the portal system, so diseases that lead to portal hypertension can lead to internal hemorrhoids.
Fecal Impaction	**Fecal impaction** occurs when fecal material is not eliminated appropriately. The retained stool forms a solid collection that impedes further passage of stool.
Encopresis	**Encopresis** is caused when chronic constipation leads to involuntary stool leakage.
Anorectal Abscess	**Anorectal abscess** is a collection of pus in the anorectal area.
Anorectal Fistula	**Anorectal fistula** is an abnormal formation of an opening in the peri-anal area, usually caused by an abscess.
Rectal Prolapse	**Rectal prolapse** occurs when rectal tissue protrudes through the anus.
Jaundice	**Jaundice** results from deposits of bile pigments in certain tissues causing a yellowish discoloration.
Biliary Colic	**Biliary colic** is pain caused by biliary tract stones.
Choledocholithiasis	**Choledocholithiasis** is the term meaning that gallstones are located in the common bile duct or the hepatic duct.
Acalculous Cholecystitis	**Acalculous cholecystitis** presents with cystitis in the absence of gallstones.
Emphysematous Cholecystitis	**Emphysematous cholecystitis** refers to cholecystitis that demonstrates gas in the wall of the gallbladder or biliary ducts.
Acute Calculous Cholecystitis	**Acute calculous cholecystitis** is an inflammation of the gallbladder because a gallstone is obstructing the cystic duct.
Gallstone Ileus	**Gallstone ileus** is intestinal obstruction caused by a gallstone in the ileum.
Cholangitis	**Cholangitis** is a bacterial infection of the biliary ducts caused by obstruction.

Term	Definition
Duct of Santorini	**Duct of Santorini** is an extra pancreatic duct that most people have, along with the duct of Wirsung.
Secretin	**Secretin** is a pancreatic enzyme high in bicarbonate that is stimulated by acidic stomach products.
Cholecystokinin-Pancreozymin	**Cholecystokinin-pancreozymin** is an enzyme released by the duodenum that is stimulated by proteins and fats. It acts on the pancreas to stimulate pancreatic enzyme release.
Grey Turner's Sign	**Grey Turner's sign** is the appearance of a bluish tinge to the flanks secondary to bleeding from acute pancreatitis.
Cullen's Sign	**Cullen's sign** is the appearance of a bluish tinge around the umbilicus secondary to bleeding from acute pancreatitis
Pseudocyst	**Pseudocyst** is a collection of pancreatic debris surrounded by granulation tissue but without a true epithelial layer.
Whipple Operation	**Whipple operation** is a pancreaticoduodenectomy to treat pancreatic cancer or other diseases.
Pancreatic Rest	**Pancreatic rest** refers to pancreatic tissue in sites other than the pancreas.
Pancreas Divisum	**Pancreas divisum** results when embryonic pancreatic tissue does not combine, causing two separate pancreatic ducts.
Annular Pancreas	**Annular pancreas** refers to a condition where embryonic tissue fails to combine and a portion of the pancreas surrounds the duodenum.
Schwachman-Diamond Syndrome	**Schwachman-Diamond syndrome** is an inherited disorder involving pancreatic insufficiency, neutropenia and growth problems.
Glisson's Capsule	**Glisson's capsule** is the connective tissue covering enveloping the liver.
Glycogenesis	**Glycogenesis** is the process the liver employs to convert glucose to glycogen for storage.
Glycogenolysis	**Glycogenolysis** is the process the liver undertakes to convert glycogen to glucose.
Gluconeogenesis	**Gluconeogenesis** is the process the liver uses to synthesize glucose.
Caput Medusae	**Caput medusae** is caused by portal hypertension leading to dilated vessels around the umbilicus.
Ascites	**Ascites** is the accumulation of fluid in the abdominal cavity.
Hepatitis	**Hepatitis** is inflammation of the liver parenchyma caused by infection, toxins, or immune reactions.
Fulminant Hepatic Failure	**Fulminant hepatic failure** is massive hepatic cell death due to an insult, such as an infection or an exposure to a toxin.
Alpha 1-Antitrypsin Deficiency	**Alpha 1 antitrypsin** or **AAT deficiency** is an inherited disease that causes a lack in the AAT enzyme, which can lead to liver and lung disease.
Biliary Atresia	**Biliary atresia** results in scarring of the biliary duct system causing cholestasis and liver damage.

Gastroenterological Procedures

Tools for Endoscopic Procedures

Endoscope

The endoscope is a flexible or rigid device used to view internal body parts, such as the esophagus, stomach, and colon. The endoscope contains a number of different channels so that instruments, air, or water can be passed and suctioning performed. A video lens and light are at the distal end, and video images are transmitted to a monitor. Some endoscopes have an eyepiece attached to the scope. Various types of endoscopes are available, including bronchoscope and colonoscope, and they come in different sizes, lengths, and flexibility.

All **endoscopes** contain the following:

- An insertion tube that is flexible and has channels for biopsy.
- A cord that is attached to the light source.
- Fiberoptic system for promulgating visual access/ video systems have camera access for television.

The **control center** which contains:

- The lens
- Controls for moving the lens
- Control valves.
- Cables for motion control.
- Channels for controlling water and air manipulation
- Biopsy channel for access via snares, forceps, brushes.

This procedure allows for visualization and biopsy of the gastrointestinal tract. It provides diagnosis and also therapy. There are a number of different endoscopes available, including the flexible endoscope, the anoscope, the proctosigmoidoscope, the flexible sigmoidoscope and the colonoscope.

Diagnostic Endoscopic Procedures

Anoscopy and Proctosigmoidoscopy

The **anoscope** aids in evaluating rectal bleeding. It is a rigid tube with a slot at the end. This is where the mucosal surface can be viewed. Evaluation of the area is done prior to inserting the scope. The patient reclines on the left with knees drawn to the chest as the lubricated anoscope is advanced. It should be lubricated and warm. The **proctosigmoidoscope** is a rigid tube with a light source used for evaluating bleeding, diarrhea, pain or extraction of a foreign body. The warmed tube is inserted to the desired point and the slowly retracted, allowing the operator to examine the mucosal surface. Complications may include perforation and bleeding.

Flexible Sigmoidoscopy

The **flexible sigmoidoscope** is more commonly used than the rigid device and is used to evaluate the rectum, the sigmoid colon and the distal end of the descending colon. The lubricated instrument is advanced up the descending colon. As the scope is slowly drawn back, the operator scrutinizes the lining of the intestines. During the procedure the operator may take biopsies, remove polyps or administer therapies such as electrocautery. The nurse must monitor vital signs, assess the comfort of the patient and evaluate for complications. Complications may include perforations and bleeding. If no complications occur, the patient may resume normal activities and a normal diet.

Colonoscopy

The **colonoscope** evaluates the gastrointestinal lining of the whole length of the large intestine. The operator advances the lubricated instrument through the large intestine. As the scope is withdrawn, the operator evaluates the lining for abnormalities. The colonoscope can also enable the operator to take biopsies, to remove polyps or to administer therapies. This procedure commonly requires sedation and anesthesia. In addition, medications to control motility may be administered. The nurse must appropriately and timely monitor vital signs and oxygenation and evaluate the status of the patient. The nurse may also need to help position the patient or to press the abdomen to help the operator maneuver the scope. Complications include perforation and bleeding.

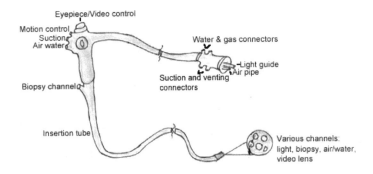

M2A Capsule Endoscopic Procedure

M2A Capsule endoscopy is a relatively new technique that allows for visualization of the small bowel. A special capsule with appropriate technology can transmit images to a receiver. Once the capsule is activated, the patient swallows the capsule. As the capsule traverses the gastrointestinal tract, it transmits images to special sensors affixed to the outside of the patient's abdomen. A recording device is worn by the patient to store the images. The patient, after not eating for six hours, swallows the capsule and cannot drink for 2 hours or eat for four hours. The process of collecting images takes approximately 8 hours, at which time the device is removed from the patient. This procedure cannot be used in patients with obstructions or electrical cardiac devices. This method offers an effective, non-invasive way to visualize the small intestine. It cannot obtain tissue or institute therapeutic maneuvers, however.

Endoscopy of an Ostomy Site

Patients with an ostomy site may need endoscopic evaluation. After draping the abdominal area around the ostomy, careful removal of the ostomy should be accomplished from top to bottom. The patient should be supine, and the operator needs to insert the endoscope from a right angle to the abdominal wall. The usual precautions concerning vital signs and oxygenation need to be taken. In addition, care should be taken to provide a tight seal between the ostomy site and the scope. After cleaning the area, the patient will need new collection apparatus.

Videoendoscopy and Endoscopic Ultrasonography

Videoendoscopy uses technology to transmit signals to a video device to display images. These video images can be seen by the entire staff and the patient. The equipment has the capability of generating photographs. The endoscope is similar to other endoscopes. **Endoscopic ultrasonography** incorporates ultrasound technology to visualize the gastrointestinal tract. The endoscope has ultrasound equipment in the tip. This procedure offers better image resolution and allows for assessing wall thickness of the various parts of the gastrointestinal tract. Some intra-abdominal organs can be seen, such as the pancreas and the gallbladder.

Endoscopic Biopsy

Endoscopic biopsy is used to obtain tissue for diagnostic purposes or to assess therapy. The scope has a biopsy channel that allows appropriate forceps to be used. At the direction of the physician, the nurse opens and closed the forceps, and the tissue sample is removed. Usually multiple samples are taken to increase the diagnostic yield. Biopsy usually is fairly superficial. With rectal suction biopsy, the tissue is suctioned and then biopsied. This allows for deeper penetration. The sample is evaluated by a pathologist. An answer can be obtained quickly, when appropriate, with a frozen section. There are disposable forceps available. Those that are re-usable must be cleaned and sterilized. Complications may include perforation and bleeding.

Fine-Needle Aspiration for Pancreatic Disease

Fine-needle aspiration of the pancreas can be accomplished through the abdominal wall under ultrasound guidance or Ct guidance. This is a fairly accurate way to diagnose pancreatic cancer. Complications may include infection. Diagnosis of pancreatic cancer can be accomplished with endoscopic ultrasound-guided fine needle aspiration. The needle is passed through the biopsy channel and it is directed to the targeted tissue by ultrasound. The recovered material is placed on a slide for evaluation. This procedure is helpful in diagnosing and in staging of cancers.

Capsule Endoscopy

Capsule endoscopy is accomplished by having the patient swallow a video capsule to visualize the bowels. The camera in the capsule sends pictures to sensors attached to the patient's body. There is a recording device attached to the patient, as well. The device enables evaluation of the small bowel.

- Once the capsule is swallowed the patient must refrain from eating for two hours. At four hours the patient can eat something light. Prior to the procedure, the patient must have nothing by mouth from midnight on.
- After 8 hours, the patient reports back with the sensors and the recorder.
- The capsule will be eliminated with stool, although it can infrequently cause obstructive symptoms. Surgery may be needed to remove the capsule.
- The patient must avoid MRI studies until the capsule is eliminated.

Obtaining Samples for Cytology

Brush cytology involves passing a small brush through the biopsy channel. The brush abrades the targeted tissue, is withdrawn and the material is applied to a slice. Sometimes the tips of the brushes are sent to the laboratory, as well. For washings, a special trap is affixed to the suction port. The endoscope allows for the suctioning of the tissues. The trap is sent for examination. The washings for an esophageal specimen can be applied via a nasogastric tube. For a gastric specimen, gastric lavage is required. For a pancreatic sample, saline is sent into the duct and aspirated back with a syringe. In the colon, after careful preparation, saline is instilled and then aspirated several minutes later.

Interventional Endoscopic Procedures

Esophagogastroduodenoscopy

The indications, contraindications. and possible adverse effects for **esophagogastroduodenoscopy (EGD)** are listed below:

- **Indications**:
  - Dysphagia
  - Odynophagia
  - Unremitting symptoms of reflux
  - Unexplained vomiting
  - Bleeding
  - Abnormalities noted by other studies, such as X-rays
  - Evaluation for cancer
  - Evaluation for response to therapy

- **Contraindications**:
  - Cardiovascular instability or shock
  - Seizures
  - Recent cardiac or pulmonary event
  - Cervical arthritis, if severe
  - Non-compliance with NPO order

- **Adverse effects**:
  - Respiratory distress
  - Cardiac distress
  - Vasovagal reaction
  - Aspiration
  - Perforation
  - Allergic reaction

EGD Procedure

Endoscopy is performed with the patient lying on the left side with the chin tucked to the midline of the chest. The lubricated scope is passed slowly through the various gastrointestinal structures, allowing time for clearing secretions and visualization. As the endoscope approaches the small bowel, the patient may report symptoms of pain or fullness. Duodenal spasm may impinge on visualization, requiring administration of a muscle relaxant. Pediatric patients are more likely to experience respiratory symptoms during the initial phase of the endoscopy. These symptoms may be alleviated by lifting the jaw forward. Throughout the endoscopy, the patient's airway should be guarded by removing secretions or other potential obstructions. Once the procedure is completed, the patient may attempt to take fluids when the gag reflex has returned.

ECRP Procedure

After the equipment has been fully tested, a side-viewing endoscope is used on the patient, who may be prone. If the patient begins on the left side, he or she must be turned to the prone position before the following step. Once the operator views the ampulla of Vater, a plastic cannula is threaded through the instrument to enter the opening in the duodenum. The cannula injects dye into the pancreatic duct or the biliary duct, depending on the operator's maneuvering. X-rays are taken, allowing depiction of the ducts to evaluate anatomy. The endoscope can also obtain tissue by biopsy or brushings. Complications of this procedure are pancreatitis and infection, along with the risk of bleeding and perforation. Some patients have an allergic reaction to the dye. Indications for an **Endoscopic retrograde cholangiopancreatography (ERCP)** include evaluation for cancer, unknown cause of pancreatitis, common bile duct stones, or unknown abdominal pain.

Sphincterotomy of the Sphincter of Oddi

Sphincterotomy is performed via ERCP to cut the muscles of the sphincter of Oddi. This may be necessary to help pass gallstones or to relieve obstructions. A side-viewing scope with appropriate cannulas is inserted into the patient. The sphincterotome should be placed superficially and then placement should be checked with radiographic evaluation. The sphincterotome is flexed and short burst of current are supplied. The passage of bile and blood signifies success, generally. The passage of stones may take longer because of edema from the procedure. Other equipment may be used to retrieve stones, if needed. A stent may need to be placed, as well.

Visualizing the Biliary Tract

Biliary tract disease can be addressed by dilatation either by ERCP or by percutaneous transhepatic cholangiography. If a stent is needed to overcome an obstruction, that can be placed, as well. A diagnostic ERCP is done to evaluate the problem and to delineate the anatomy. A guidewire is passed and then a silicone sprayed balloon. The balloon is inflated according to the manufacturer's directions. The inflation can be repeated. Sometimes a stent can be placed after the inflations are completed. Pancreatitis is the most common complication. The bile ducts may sustain some injury, as well.

Endoscopic Variceal Ligation Procedures

Endoscopic variceal ligation or EVL involves placing bands or rings around the varix or hemorrhoid. Several instruments are available, and the manufacturer's directions should be carefully followed. The varix or hemorrhoid is sucked into the ligating device and the ligature is placed around the tissue. The suction is then released. Although the band device is more expensive, it offers some advantages over the O-ring applicator, particularly the ability to perform multiple banding steps with one endoscopic insertion. Both procedures result in less pain for the patient and are less likely to cause strictures.

Ablation of Cancerous Obstruction with Bipolar Probe

A guidewire is passed through an endoscope with guidance by fluoroscopy, if possible. Then the endoscope is removed. Dilators may be needed to allow for passage of the probe to the distal area of the obstruction. Current is applied in a proximal pattern until the most proximal site is treated. Endoscopy is repeated to ascertain the effectiveness of therapy. The patient must be monitored afterwards and kept NPO. Some patients may complain of dysphagia for a day after the procedure. Another endoscopy is performed in two days to determine the efficacy of the treatment and to assess if another course of therapy is needed.

Injection Therapy

Injection therapy is used to treat esophageal varices that are bleeding. The operator injects a substance in or around a targeted variceal abnormality to stop any bleeding. The endoscopist passes an endoscope, preferably double channeled to allow for suction, and then introduces the needle assembly. The patient must be medically stable and cooperative. Emergency therapy should be available at all times. When the bleeding site is located, the needle is injected into the targeted site. The chosen agent is injected at the physician's direction. Once completed, the needle assembly can be discarded according to the sharps protocol.

Removal of Foreign Bodies in Gastrointestinal Tract

Removal of foreign bodies can be accomplished with endoscopy or surgery. In the vast majority of cases, foreign bodies pass through the gastrointestinal tract without intervention, however. Foreign bodies tend to get lodged where there is narrowing, like the LES. Removal must move forward for foreign bodies that are sharp to prevent bleeding or perforation. Also, batteries need to be removed quickly to prevent caustic injury from the contents of the battery. In the case of drug packet foreign bodies, surgery is the best treatment to avoid overdose and/or death. Foreign bodies in the stomach that are larger than 2 centimeters need to be acted upon, as do any stomach foreign bodies that do not pass within 2 weeks. Similarly, foreign bodies that persist in the duodenum for 6 days need to be removed.

To **endoscopically remove a foreign body** from the esophagus, the operator must have a firm hold on the object. This will ensure that the object is not inappropriately dropped where it can interfere with respiration. If the object is sharp, the sharpened end should be pointed away from the direction of removal. Sometimes an overtube or a hood is placed over the endoscope to protect the mucosal surface of the esophagus, as well as the airway. Impacted food can be pushed into the stomach by using dilators, if needed. For objects that lodge in the large intestine can be removed by colonoscopy, using forceps or retrieval nets. Objects in the sigmoid or rectal area can be removed by an appropriate scope, such as a sigmoidoscope, a proctoscope or an anoscope.

Gastrointestinal Specimens

Processing and Handling of Gastrointestinal Specimens

Processing and handling for **gastrointestinal specimens** includes:

- *Gastric aspirate*: Place aspirate (at least 1 mL) in gastric aspirate tube with bicarbonate or specimen cup for transportation to the laboratory. If no bicarbonate is in the container, the sample should be neutralized with bicarbonate within 30 minutes.
- *Duodenal aspirate*: Place specimen (at least 2 mL) in sterile centrifuge tube and transport to the laboratory immediately for examination within 60 minutes of collection.
- *Gastric and rectal biopsy specimens*: Tissue specimen is placed in a sterile container with a preservative, such as formalin and labeled with identifying information and the location from which the sample was obtained. The specimen undergoes a gross examination as well as microscopic. The sample may be preserved in paraffin wax and cut into slices which are placed on a slide and examined microscopically. If results are required quickly (such as when the surgeon is waiting to continue surgery), a frozen section may be done.

Fecal samples should be directly collected or placed in a clean container and further processed according to the type of testing that will be carried out.

- *Culture*: Place in liquid transport media with preservative, such as orange Cary-Blair container, and test within 14 days. Unpreserved stool must be tested within 2 hours.
- *& P (Giardia and Cryptosporidium):* Place is liquid transport media (as above) and test within 14 days. Unpreserved stool may be refrigerated at 2° to 8° C but must be tested within 72 hours.
- *& P (other):* Place in Parasep SF (green) containing preservative, such as Alcor Fix) within 1 hour of collection for testing up to 9 months. May be stored at room temperature or under refrigeration. Unpreserved stool must be tested within 2 hours.
- *WBC*: Unpreserved stool specimen must be tested within 2 hours.
- *Occult blood*: Smear sample of stool onto card, which must be tested within 14 days.
- *Clostridium difficile*: Place unpreserved semi-liquid/liquid stool in container and submit immediately for testing within 24 hours at room temperature or within 5 days if refrigerated at 2° to 8° C.
- *Rotavirus*: Place unpreserved specimen in container and submit immediately for testing.

Tools for Non-Endoscopic Procedures

Probes Used in Non-Endoscopic Procedures

Probes are thin solid or flexible instruments or catheters used to explore or assess wounds, body cavities, and body organs. Various probes used in non-endoscopic procedures include:

- *Ultrasound probe*: May help to identify problems in blood flow to the GI system, and may help in diagnosis of gall stones and liver disease, such as scarring indicating cirrhosis.
- *Eyed probe*: Has a small "eye" or opening at one end which can carry ligatures. This 6-inch probe can be used to help determine the size and depth of fistulas or cavities.
- *Esophageal pH probe*: A thin probe is inserted nasally and into the esophagus and attached to a monitor that continually assesses acidity, usually for a 24-hour period, to aid in the diagnosis of acid reflux. A 48-hour probe involves attaching a small monitor by catheter to the distal portion of the esophagus. This monitor sends acidity recordings wirelessly to a recorder worn on the body and automatically detaches and passes through the intestinal tract after 48 hours.

Use of Ligature in Non-Endoscopic Procedures

The use of **ligature** in non-endoscopic procedures includes:

- *Rubber band ligation*: Used primarily for first- and second-degree hemorrhoids and involves placing a band about the base of the hemorrhoid and leaving it in place to cut off the blood supply to the hemorrhoid. Over the next 7 days or so, the tissue sloughs off. While slight bleeding and mild discomfort is common, there is also a small risk of severe bleeding and sepsis.
- *Ligation of intersphincteric fistula tract (LIFT):* This method of ligation for fistula-in-ano is used primarily for trans-sphincteric fistulae and involves incision to identify the intersphincteric fistula tract, ligation and removal of the tract, curetting of the tract, and suturing at the external sphincter muscle. This procedure prevents fecal material from contaminating the tract and allows it to heal, preserving the sphincter. Success rates vary and range from 57% to 94% and some fistula recur, but are usually less severe.

Diagnostic Non-Endoscopic Procedures

Manometry

Equipment

Esophageal manometry assesses pressures within the esophagus and evaluates motility and coordination of the muscular activity of the esophagus. This technique is useful if other diseases causing the symptoms have been ruled out, if the information would add to the knowledge needed to treat the patient, and in placing pH probes. The instrument is a tube that includes a pressure transducer to reflect pressures as an audible and recordable signal. It also houses a water-perfused catheter or a solid-state probe to measure the pressures and activities. Prior to using, the equipment must be checked and the patient evaluated. The catheter is inserted, and the patient is told to swallow to help the tube pass. Once the tube is in the stomach, appropriate measurements can be obtained. Afterwards, the catheters are rinsed with detergent, rinsed and dried, and sterilized via ethylene oxide. If a solid-state probe was used, this is subjected to high level disinfection alone.

Manometry Evaluation of Esophagus

To assess the LES, the catheter is pulled back through the LES. If done rapidly, the LES location can be determined. Pulling more slowly gives a fuller picture of the functioning of the LES. When the catheter enters the thoracic cavity, the tracing goes down; this is called the respiration inversion point. **To assess the esophageal body**, the catheter is stationed so that its ports are located throughout the length of the esophagus. The patient performs swallowing to allow the ports to assess the coordination and activity of the muscles of the esophagus. Normally, the movement is a coordinated and progressive wave of activity. Abnormalities in strength and coordination can be detected. **To assess the UES**, the manometric ports evaluate the pressure with swallowing.

Provocative Testing

Provocative testing is used to help determine the origin of chest pain, assuming heart disease has been ruled out. The **Bernstein test** uses a nasogastric tube or a manometric tube to drip alternating solutions of saline and dilute acid into the esophagus. The patient is asked to indicate when pain occurs. **Edrophonium testing** also helps elucidate non-cardiac chest pain. After a manometric exam, a catheter is inserted; the catheter has several portals. Edrophonium, a cholinesterase inhibitor, is altered with saline intravenously. The edrophonium promotes muscle contractions. If this replicates the patient's pain, it is a positive test.

Diagnosis of Esophageal Diseases

Manometry is used to diagnose achalasia, which results from loss of esophageal motility and increased LES tone. The instrument should be passed through the LES so that the sphincter tone and pressure can be determines. The LES may have insufficient relaxation or may have a very short period of relaxation. For diffuse esophageal spasm, the manometry reveals concomitant smooth muscle contractions towards the LES region. For nutcracker esophagus, the manometry reveals amplified contractions that may be prolonged. These patients are likely to have a reaction to edrophonium. Manometry can also assess LES tension and other motility abnormalities. Diabetics, for example, are prone to esophageal motility disorders. For esophageal reflux, patients may have some manometric abnormalities, but pH monitoring is more useful.

Other Uses

Gastroduodenal manometry is useful in assessing motility disorders in the stomach and small intestines. It can help in the diagnosis of gastroparesis and gastric arrythmias. **Small bowels** can be evaluated for motility disorders or dumping syndromes. The manometric apparatus is inserted over a guidewire and is able to assess measurements at the antrum, the duodenum and the small bowel. The **sphincter of Oddi** can be evaluated for motility disorders, as well as stenosis. This can be done via ERCP. A catheter, equipped with manometry, is passed up the biliary tract, and the manometer is pulled back to assess pressures.

Anorectal Manometry

Anorectal manometry is useful in investigating, constipation, incontinence, connective tissue disease, Hirschsprung's disease and Chagas' disease. The instrument is composed of a balloon, and two sensors; one for the internal sphincter and one for the external sphincter. The balloon is inflated and then sphincter responses are assessed. Normally the internal sphincter should relax as the bowel distends; the external sphincter tightens. Some health practitioners have used anorectal manometry as a form of biofeedback for patients with incontinence problems due to other causes such as trauma or multiple sclerosis. The patient may be able to learn appropriate reactions to the stimulation from rectal distention.

Liver Biopsy Procedures

Percutaneous liver biopsy can be done to diagnose liver disease and to stage cancers. If the patient is determined to be a good candidate, he/she should be educated and evaluated prior to the procedure. An IV should be placed and vital signs documented. After the skin is carefully cleaned, the layers overlying the liver are anesthetized. A small incision is made and the needle, which is attached to a syringe, is inserted. The syringe has sterile saline for flushing the needle. Liver tissue is aspirated through the needle and then placed in saline or formalin. In some cases, the biopsy is guided by ultrasound or CT. After the procedure, the wound must be damped for 2 hours, accompanied by bed rest for six to eight hours. The patient must be monitored for bleeding, peritonitis, infection or other signs of complications.

Radiographic Studies of Gastrointestinal Tract

Radiographic studies of the gastrointestinal tract are used to evaluate anatomy and to look for pathology. These tests are often better tolerated, but the diagnostic yield is not as good as endoscopic procedures. **Barium sulfate** is the commonly used contrast medium, allowing for X-ray and fluoroscopic studies. Since the Barium may interfere with other kinds of studies, it should be done after those are completed. The patient should be advised that stools will be lighter colored, but this should be completed in a few days. It is important that the patient eliminate the Barium so they do not develop constipation. **Radiographs of the pancreas, the gallbladder and the biliary tree** are done using an iodine-based contrast medium. Some patients are allergic to the medium.

Imaging Studies to Evaluate the Biliary System

The following are **imaging studies for evaluating the biliary system**:

- **Magnetic Resonance Cholangiopancreatography** evaluate the biliary system and the pancreatic ducts, avoiding an ERCP. The patient is given a contrast medium, gadolinium.
- **Percutaneous transhepatic cholangiography** visualizes the biliary system by passing a skinny needle through the liver until a bile duct is penetrated. Iodine contrast medium is then added so that the system can be evaluated.

- 57 -

- **Abdominal ultrasound** uses sound waves to visualize abdominal organs. A transducer traverses the patient's abdomen, converting the reflected sound waves to images.
- **Oral cholecystography** studies the biliary system by having the patient ingest pills with contrast medium. 10-14 hours later, the films are taken.

Uses of Scintigraphy in the Gastrointestinal Tract

Scintigraphy uses radioisotopes to assess anatomy and pathology. **Hepatic Scintigraphy** is used to study the liver. The Kupfer cells absorb the radioisotope; abnormal structures without Kupffer cells are not visualized. It is used to assess metastatic disease, hepatocellular disease or other infiltrating diseases. **Biliary scintigraphy** introduces a radioisotope that is taken up by liver cells and then passed into the bile system so that the biliary system can be visualized. Gastric emptying can be assessed by using a radioisotope to label food that is ingested by the patient. The scanner follows the course of the labeled food. **Scintigraphic scanning** may be used to evaluate gastrointestinal bleeding. Labeled red blood cells are given to the patient and scanning follows their course through the circulatory system. This same technique can be used to label white blood cells to look for inflammation.

Secretion Studies of the Gastrointestinal Tract

Pancreatic stimulation requires placement of a duodenal tube. The pancreas is stimulated by secretin and cholecystokinin. Secretions are evaluated to determine if there is exocrine insufficiency or other diseases. Gastric analysis requires that a tube be placed along the greater curvature and reaches the most dependent area of the stomach. Basal acid secretions are obtained and then secretions resulting from stimulation by the enzyme pentagastrin are measured. This can determine if there is too much acid, as in Zollinger-Ellison syndrome, or not enough acid, as in achlorhydria. 24-hour pH monitoring allows for assessment of acid levels over a long period. This assesses esophageal reflux or evaluates chest pain. The pH probe is passed though the esophagus to just above the LES. The pH levels are recorded, as are patient symptoms and activities.

Liver Function Tests

The following are **tests of liver function**:

- **Serum bilirubin** is produced by the liver and secreted with bile. It can be measured in the blood. If there is an excess of bilirubin in the blood, it may indicate a blockage to bile flow, an inability of the liver to process bile, or an overproduction of bilirubin.
- **Alkaline phosphatase** is an enzyme that can be measured in the blood. This is a measure of the excretory functioning of the liver. Many tissues have alkaline phosphatase, but there are high amounts in the liver and bone. Alkaline phosphatase is elevated in obstruction of the biliary tree, metastatic disease and fatty infiltration.
- **Serum aminotransferases** are aspartate aminotransferase or AST and alanine aminotransferase or ALT. These enzymes, made in the liver, assess cellular integrity. ALT is especially elevated from abnormalities due to viruses or drugs. It is less elevated in alcoholic liver disease.
- **Gamma glutamyl transferase or GGT** is used to differentiate bone alkaline phosphatase, since its concomitant elevation indicates that the elevation in alkaline phosphatase comes from the liver.

Evaluation for a Coagulopathy

The ability of blood to clot depends on a number of different interactions, many of which can be affected by gastrointestinal tract diseases. **Prothrombin becomes thrombin to promote clotting.** If vitamin K is not adequately absorbed in the intestine, the level of prothrombin may be decreased. Diseases that disrupt liver function can lead to decreased levels. The conversion of prothrombin to thrombin involves a cascade of reactions involving factors, some of which are made in the liver. **Prothrombin time or PT** is used to assess the speed with which blood clots. Increased clotting times reflect liver disease, malnutrition, or certain genetic diseases. The **activated partial thromboplastin time or APTT** is another test to measure blood clotting. The **International Normalized Ratio or INR** is derived by comparing the patient's PT with the mean level of a large group of people.

Blood Tests for Viral Hepatitis

Hepatitis can be caused by a number of viruses. **Hepatitis B surface antigen or HBsAg** can be detected in carriers, as well as in patients with acute or chronic infection with Hepatitis B. **Hepatitis B core antibody or HBcAB** is found in acute and post infectious cases. Immunoglobulin M would be needed to determine active infection; Immunoglobulin G denotes post infection. **Hepatitis B e antigen or HBeAg** indicates a significant infection, but the patient is no longer contagious. **Hepatitis A antibody or HAVAB** is detected in ongoing infections and in those recovered from infection. **Hepatitis C is detected by finding anti-HCV** in the patient. However, in patients with an acute hepatitis C infection may not produce antibodies for a number of months. Hepatitis D only infects those with hepatitis B infection.

Use of Urinalysis in Gastrointestinal Diseases

Urine bilirubin measures the amount of direct bilirubin; elevations suggest liver or biliary disease. **Urine urobilinogen**, when elevated, reflects the inability of liver cells to handle urobilinogen, which is produced from intestinal breakdown of bilirubin. **Schilling test** is a test to measure the ability of the small bowel to absorb vitamin B12. Radioisotopes are administered orally with and without intrinsic factor. B12 is also given intravenously. Assessing the various amounts of radioisotopes in a 24-hour urine can suggest the cause of vitamin B12 malabsorption.

Fecal Tests

The following are tests that can be done on feces:

- **Fecal urobilinogen** can be decreased in biliary obstruction, causing clay colored stools.
- **Fecal occult blood** indicates gastrointestinal bleeding. Three samples must be assessed. A small sample is placed on a hem occult card and treated with a reagent. If the sample becomes blue, it indicates blood. Certain foods and vitamins can lead to false positives.
- **Fecal fat** is assessed as a measure of malabsorption and excess fetal fat or steatorrhea. Stools should be collected over 72 hours, and the amount of fat in the stool is compared to the fat ingested during that time by the patient.
- **Fecal chymotrypsin** levels can indicate insufficiency of pancreatic exocrine function.
- **Stools** can be collected to assess for ova and parasites, white blood cells and organisms. The sample can also be cultured.

H. pylori Infection

Infection with *H. pylori* is associated with peptic ulcer disease. Treatment of the organism may alleviate ulcer disease. Detection of *H. pylori* disease can be done with blood tests, breath tests, stool tests and biopsy specimens. The urea breath tests are done by having the patient drink a urea solution with labeled carbon. *H. pylori* breaks down the urea, the carbon is absorbed and then the carbon is eliminated through the lungs. The carbon-13 blood test measures antibodies to *H. pylori*. *H. pylori* Stool antigen test or HpSA test detects the *H. pylori* antigen in the stool.

Interventional Non-Endoscopic Procedures

Esophageal Dilatation

Esophageal dilatation is performed to treat abnormalities that result in patients having difficulty eating. The procedure can be done on a daily basis, if needed. Those who cannot cooperate have had a recent major cardiac or pulmonary event, or have a coagulopathy should not undergo esophageal dilatation. Complications of dilatation may include perforation, bleeding, aspiration or infection. Perforation needs to be identified quickly. That may require X-rays looking for inappropriate collection of air or lung abnormalities. Surgery may be necessary.

Sheer-Force Dilators

Bougies are one kind of sheer-force dilator that can be used. These are made of rubber or silicone and are weighted with mercury or tungsten. These are also called the Hurst or Maloney dilatators. The Maloney dilators are tapered; the Hurst dilators are rounded. These dilators are used to treat strictures, rings or webs, diffuse esophageal spasm and scleroderma. The other sheer-force dilator is the **Savary-Gilliard or American dilators.** These are made of polyvinyl chloride. The dilator is placed over a guidewire that was positioned by endoscopy. These kinds of dilatators are used to treat esophageal strictures or to place a stent.

Bougienage

The lubricated bougie is passed into the esophagus. When the narrowing is encountered, the physician carefully pushes the instrument forward. Each bougie must be carefully inspected to be sure it is in good condition. Cleaning the bougie requires use of an enzymatic cleaner and to fulfill disinfection instructions supplied by the manufacturer. The instrument is then rinsed, completely dried and stored in a horizontal position. Rubber bougies need to be removed quickly from cleaning solutions to prevent damage. Silicone bougies must be cleaned with mild soap and water.

Nursing Duties During Esophageal Dilatation

The nurse must ascertain that the patient has been NPO for at least six hours, that the medical history is accurate, that the patient understands the procedure and why it's being done, remove dentures, establish basic vital signs and start an IV. The nurse must help the patient to maintain his/her position to reduce the risk of perforation. Use of a guidewire requires the nurse to inspect it and to hold the loose end as the physician passes it. The nurse must keep the physician informed of vital signs, signs of complications and evidence of blood on the equipment or in any secretions. The nurse may need to apply suction to help the doctor or to provide comfort for the patient.

Hydrostatic Balloons

Hydrostatic balloons can be used to dilate strictures in the esophagus, the pylorus, the duodenum, the rectum or the left colon. It can also be used for biliary tract strictures and to treat certain food impactions. Hydrostatic balloons are filled with either water or dilute radiopaque dye. The through-the-scope balloons go through the biopsy channel of the endoscope and inflate to a diameter of 4 to 25 millimeters. The over-the-guide wire balloons can be inflated to a diameter of 4 to 40 millimeters. The balloon must be checked for leaks before they are used. Once inserted to the appropriate location, the balloon can be inflated according to orders or to manufacturer's instructions. The inflated balloon remains for a short period and is then deflated. This may be repeated, if the patient tolerates it. When the balloon is removed it must be inspected for blood. After its use, the balloon is cleaned, disinfected and stored according to the manufacturer's instructions.

Pneumatic Balloons

Pneumatic balloons are used to stretch the LES. This is needed in patients with achalasia. This maneuver causes the circular muscle to tear, reducing the pressure. Pneumatic balloons may also be a second line treatment for esophageal rings that have not responded to bougienage. Many physicians prefer to have the patient observed over 24 hours. The patient is instructed to maintain a liquid diet the day before the procedure. Review of the procedure should include information that there may be pain, and there is medication available to help alleviate discomfort. The patient is under conscious sedation. The balloon is passed over a guidewire and then inflated when in place. Fluoroscopic evaluation should accompany the procedure. The esophagus must be cleared as needed. The physician should be notified if the dilator has blood when removed. Complications may include perforation, bleeding or aspiration. Some physicians do a follow-up contrast study to check for perforations or tears.

Electrocautery or Electrocoagulation

Electrocautery or electrocoagulation employs an electrical current to a source of bleeding to coagulate tissue in order to stop bleeding. The instruments used are electrical surgical units. Care must be taken to ensure that all cords and connections are intact; the instrument should be tested prior to the procedure. For the upper gastrointestinal tract, a diagnostic endoscopy should locate the source and then therapy should be applied. There should be no blood in the stomach. For the colon, the bowel must be cleaned for proper visualization and to eliminate gases that might explode. The patient should be medically stable, and the nurse should educate and assure the patient. Also, the nurse must monitor the patient. Complications may include burns, bleeding, perforation and explosion.

Monopolar Electrocoagulation

Monopolar electrocoagulation applies current from the device to the local site. The patient has a grounding pad placed on the skin over a well vascularized, non-boney area. The subsequent heat generated leads to coagulation of the tissue. Soft, disposable pads provide the best contact. Patients need to be warned not to touch anything metal during the intervention. It is important to avoid current leakage, which can lead to burns to the patient or burns to the operator. The nurse needs to attach the grounding pad appropriately, wear rubber gloves, avoid touching the patient during the intervention, and be certain the patient does not touch metal.

Bipolar Electrosurgery and Bipolar Electrocoagulation

Bipolar electrosurgery requires greater expertise, but provides therapy as effectively as monopolar electrosurgery with less mucosal damage. **Bipolar electrocoagulation** does not use a grounding pad. Instead, it uses a bipolar probe, which handles the current. Water can be issued from the scope to clear the targeted area. Bipolar electrocoagulation offers some advantages over monopolar electrocoagulation. There is more control over the penetration depth so that perforations are less likely. The effect of bipolar electrocoagulation has less effect on surrounding tissue since it does not travel as far. This form of therapy can also provide the advantage of tamponading a vessel prior to coagulation. Complications include perforation, bleeding and ulcerations.

Laser Therapy

Laser therapy can be used to treat gastrointestinal bleeding or to treat obstructing or abnormal lesions. Usually lasers using **Neodymium (Yttrium-Aluminum-Garnet or YAG Lasers)** are operated by endoscopists, although some use Argon lasers. The laser transmits light energy to the targeted area by being passed through an endoscope. To avoid damaging the endoscope, appropriate scopes should be employed and treatments should be delivered when the laser is away from the scope. **Photocoagulation** results from heat at 60 C and results in tissue coagulation. Photovaporization occurs at 100 C and is used to destroy or cut tissue. After testing the laser, the preferred two-channel endoscope is inserted into the patient. The double channel allows for removal of generated gases. Everyone needs protective eye gear and a laser mask. Appropriate warning signs need to be in place to prevent inadvertent exposure. Complication may include bleeding, perforation, ulceration, fistula formation or stricture formation.

Laser Therapy for Gastrointestinal Tumors

Laser therapy for gastrointestinal tumors focuses on controlling bleeding and obstructive symptoms, although curative therapy can sometimes by accomplished. The laser is passed through the endoscope, and it begins therapy on the target tissue closest to the lumen. The following treatments are administered in circles around the initial target area until, but not including, the wall of the gastrointestinal tract. Many operators prefer to use photocoagulation rather than vaporization because less smoke is generated. This form of therapy should be reserved for those who have no alternative for achieving a cure. Esophageal tumors may require several treatments to achieve results. Rectal tumors can often be done on an outpatient basis. If the tumor encroaches on the anus, appropriate medication needs to be administered because this may cause pain during treatment.

Photodynamic Therapy

Photodynamic therapy or PDT uses a red-light laser to treat abnormalities, such as dysplasia, Barrett's esophagus or superficial adenocarcinomas. The patient is given a medication beforehand that concentrates in the abnormal tissue. The medication makes the tissue sensitive to light. The red-light laser destroys the targeted tissues. Patients must avoid sunlight for a little more than a month. Although there are some side effects, such as nausea, swallowing difficulties or pain, this treatment offers the advantage of not having to use heat in the treatment intervention.

Sclerotherapy

Sclerotherapy involves injecting a sclerosing agent into varices to stop bleeding. It can also be used to control bleeding from hemorrhoids. The function is to destroy the vessel causing the bleeding.

Commonly, one of three sclerosing materials is used: Scleromate, Sotradecol or Ethamolin. The latter is the least likely to cause ulcers. Some patients can manifest an allergic reaction to these agents. If the patient is actively bleeding, visualization is difficult. Bleeding can be tempered by using vasopressin or balloon tamponade. For those bleeding, the initial treatment should be administered just above the point of origin and then to either side of the initial injection site. It is also important to treat the area below the bleeding varix. Complications may include perforation, ulceration or stricture formation.

Esophageal-Gastric Tamponade

Esophageal-gastric tamponade allows the operator to tamponade bleeding areas by applying pressure to those areas with tubes. This procedure is usually reserved for hemorrhaging that has not responded to other therapies. After determining that the equipment is in good working order, it is inserted, and then its placement is checked by X-ray. The gastric balloon is slowly inflated once the stomach has been cleared. This is pulled back to exert pressure on the lumen to provide tamponade. If this does not stop the bleeding, the esophageal balloon should be used. The gastric and esophageal balloons can be inflated together if the source of the bleed is esophageal. The tamponading can be discontinued after 24 hours if the bleeding has stopped. Complications may include rupture, aspiration or tissue necrosis.

Nasogastric Tubes

There are many **nasogastric tubes** available for use. Function of the tube must be considered in terms of how it would be used. Suction and feedings may require a larger bore tube. Those tubes most commonly used are the Levin tube the Salem sump tube, the extended use nasogastric feeding tube, the Moss tube and the Compat tube. Determining that the patient can tolerate the tube is important, including prior surgeries or fractures. A lubricated tube is inserted in one of the nostrils, having the patient put chin to chest upon entering the area above the trachea. Care should be taken to avoid cannulating the respiratory system. Confirming proper placement may be ascertained by passing air through the tube and listening for appropriate sounds via the stethoscope. The tube should be anchored for stability.

The Levin tube works like a vacuum, sticking to the stomach mucosal surface. Therefore, constant suction should not be applied. **The Salem sump tube** has two lumens, one for suction and drainage and one for venting. The venting channel does not allow a vacuum to form. The **extended-use nasogastric feeding tube** can remain in place for about a month. The **Moss tube** has two lumens with ports for balloons, duodenal feelings and aspiration. The **Compat tube** has a port for decompressions and drainage. This port can also be used to give medications.

PEG Tube

Percutaneous endoscopic gastrostomy (PEG), used for tube feedings, involves intubation of the esophagus with the endoscope and insertion of a sheathed needle with a guidewire through the abdomen and stomach wall so that a catheter can be fed down the esophagus, snared, and pulled out through the opening where the needle was inserted and secured. The PEG tube should not be secured to the abdomen until the PEG is fully healed, which usually takes 2 to 4 weeks, because tension caused by taping the tube against the abdomen may cause the tract to change shape and direction. The tract should be straight to facilitate insertion and removal of catheters. Once the tract has healed, the original PEG tube can generally be replaced with a balloon gastrostomy tube. External stabilizing devices can be applied to the skin to hold the tube in place but should be placed 1 to 2 cm above the skin surface to prevent excessive tension that may result in buried bumper syndrome (BBS) in which the internal fixation device becomes lodged in the mucosal lining of the gastric wall, resulting in ulceration.

Transjugular Intrahepatic Portosystemic Shunt

Transjugular intrahepatic portosystemic or TIPS shunts can alleviate portal hypertension without surgery. This is a new procedure, and long-term outcomes have, therefore, not been assessed. The right hepatic vein is accessed via a wire from the right internal jugular vein. A sheath is then passed into the portal vein and an angioplasty balloon is inflated. A stent is placed from the hepatic vein to the portal vein. This allows shunting of the blood to the inferior vena cava. Complications may include perforation, bleeding, infection and subsequent blockage of the stent.

Polypectomy

Polyps can be removed by a polypectomy snare or by hot biopsy forceps. Different polyps require different equipment and techniques. Some polyps need to be ensnared, some need to be removed in pieces, others are efficiently removed with just a hot biopsy forceps. For multiple polyps, the operator may have to make several passes. Once the polyp is removed, it is examined for the presence of cancer. The operator may re-insert the scope to assess the excised area. Complications may include bleeding, perforation, explosion from gases, or burns from the equipment. Sometimes bleeding can be managed with immediate treatment with the available equipment. The operator may ensnare the area, holding it until bleeding is stopped. Also, electrocoagulation, treatment with a heater probe, or injection therapy may be used.

Non-Invasive Treatments for Gallstones

Extracorporeal shock-wave lithotripsy or ESWL uses shock waves to break up stones instead of undergoing a cholecystectomy. The results are better in those with less than 3 stones, adequate gallbladder function and thin habitus. This method is often used with dissolution of gallstones. There have been occurrences of obstruction requiring subsequent ERCP. Another method to deal with stones is the use of the pulsed-dye laser. The laser is fired at a point in contact with the quartz wire, fragmenting the stone. This method is more rapid and can treat a larger number of stones than ESWL.

Surgical Interventions for Esophageal Disorders

GERD that does not respond to medical management may be treated by surgery. The most common procedure, **a Nissen fundoplication,** involved wrapping the stomach around the lower esophagus to act as a sphincter. This can be done through laparotomy or laparoscopy. There are also some investigational procedures that are promising. **Achalasia may require surgical intervention**. **Heller's myotomy** is the usual surgical procedure. The esophagus is approaches from without and cuts are made to the lower musculature of the esophagus. This causes relaxation of the LES. Since reflux symptoms are a common complication of this procedure, another procedure to treat the development of those symptoms is performed, as well. **Esophageal cancer** in the distal 2/3 of the esophagus can be performed for localized disease. Through an abdominal incision, the diseased area is removed. The esophagus is reattached to the stomach. Enteral feeding through a gastrostomy tube can be done during the acute recovery period.

Surgical Procedures for Gastric Disorders

Hiatal hernias may be repaired surgically by reducing the hernia and tacking the anatomy into place. **Obesity** can be addressed through surgical intervention, either vertical banded gastroplasty

- 64 -

or Roux-en-Y gastric bypass. In the banded procedure, staples stretch from the fundus to the upper part of the lesser curvature. This cuts off access of food to the rest of the stomach. With the Roux-en-Y, the fundus-lesser curvature pouch is created, but also the jejunum is fixed to the pouch. The duodenum is then fixed to the jejunum. **Peptic ulcer disease** can be treated surgically with Billroth I, Billroth II, vagotomy or a combination of these procedures. A **perforated ulcer** can be treated with suturing acutely, followed at a later time with one of the procedures mentioned for ulcer disease therapy. **Hypertrophic pyloric stenosis** can be treated with pyloromyotomy, cutting the muscles around the pylorus. **Gastric cancer** can be removed by surgery. If the entire stomach must be removed, the esophagus is attached to the jejunum.

Surgical Procedures for Pancreatic Disorders

Pancreatic cancer can be treated with surgery. The intervention is called Whipple's procedure and is technically a pancreaticoduodenectomy. The surgery removes half the stomach, the duodenum, the proximal jejunum, the gallbladder, the distal biliary tree and the head, neck and uncinate process of the pancreas. A modified form of this procedure does not remove the stomach and upper part of the duodenum. With added radiation therapy and chemotherapy, outcomes have improved in recent years. For intractable or life-threatening **pancreatitis**, pancreaticoduodenectomy may be attempted.

Surgical Procedures for Disorders of the Colon

Hirschsprung's disease is treated by removing the affected part of the bowel. **Inflammatory bowel disease** may require surgery for control of symptoms or complications. Removal of the colon is done with connection of the ileum to the rectum, if the rectum is clear. If not, an ileostomy will need to be accommodated. **Colon cancer** can be treated by surgery. Removal of the affected bowel can be performed. **Colon perforation** can be treated by closure and rinsing of the abdominal cavity. Part of the colon may need to be removed in some cases.

Important Terms

Term	Definition
Gastrointestinal Manometry	**Gastrointestinal manometry** is used to assess pressures and motility in the gastrointestinal tract.
Respiration Inversion Point	**Respiration inversion point** is the movement of the manometric catheter from the abdominal cavity into the thoracic cavity.
Scleroderma	**Scleroderma** is a connective tissue disease that leads to loss of esophageal motility because of absent muscle contraction.
Bernstein Test	**Bernstein test** is a provocative test using exogenous acid exposure to reproduce chest pain.
Anorectal Manometry	**Anorectal manometry** assesses the response of the internal and external sphincters to the stimulus of bowel distention.
Systemic Amyloidosis	**Systemic amyloidosis** is the abnormal condition of the buildup of amyloid in the intestinal wall.
Hot Biopsy Forceps	**Hot biopsy forceps** are for electrocoagulating tissue for those at increased risk of bleeding.
Rectal Culture	**Rectal culture** is accomplished by swabbing the rectal area looking for infectious disease.
Carey Capsule	**Carey capsule** is equipment that allows for small bowel biopsy.
Crosby Capsule	**Crosby capsule** is equipment that allows for small bowel biopsy.

Term	Definition
Frozen Section Biopsy	**Frozen section** is a biopsy that is immediately mounted and examined for quick results.
Brush Cytology	**Brush cytology** involves passing a tiny brush through the biopsy channel.
Barium Swallow	**Barium swallow** is a study in which a patient swallows the radiopaque contrast so that the esophagus can be evaluated.
Upper Gastrointestinal Series	**Upper gastrointestinal series** or **UGI** with small bowel follow through allows the evaluation of the gastrointestinal tract through the small bowel by using radiopaque Barium.
Enteroclysis	**Enteroclysis** allows for injection Barium through a tube to evaluate the small bowel.
Barium Enema	**Barium enema** used radiopaque Barium to assess the colon.
Arteriography	**Arteriography** or **angiography** is a test in which arteries are injected with contrast medium to assess bleeding, trauma or vascular abnormalities.
Computed Tomography	**Computed tomography** or **CT** is an imaging study that computes the different densities of tissues to make an image.
Biliary Drainage Studies	**Biliary drainage studies** require that a tube be passed into the duodenum and then the gallbladder is stimulated to contract. Secretions are collected and examined.
Hemoglobin	**Hemoglobin** reflects the pigment responsible for carrying oxygen in the red blood cell.
Hematocrit	**Hematocrit** defines the percent volume of red blood cells to the whole blood.
Bleeding Time	**Bleeding time** is measure of platelet function. The time it takes a patient to clot after a cut can be timed.
Platelets	**Platelets**, manufactured in the bone marrow, are blood cells that help in clotting blood. If they are low, the patient will have a tendency to bleed.
Serum D-Xylose Test	**Serum d-xylose test** assesses the ability of the small intestine, particularly the upper small bowel, to absorb necessary substances.
Glucose Tolerance Test	**Glucose tolerance test** assesses a patient's ability to respond to a glucose challenge. Abnormal responses suggest diabetes.
Serum Cholesterol	**Serum cholesterol** is measured for a number of reasons. Elevated levels are associated with increased cardiac disease and may be caused by certain diseases, including gastrointestinal diseases.
Carcinoembryonic Antigen	**Carcinoembryonic antigen** levels are elevated with certain forms of cancer or inflammatory diseases.
Breath Tests	**Breath tests** require the measurement of exhaled gases after the ingestion of a labeled substance.
Bougienage	**Bougienage** is the procedure to dilate the esophagus by using a weighted bougie to push through an esophageal narrowing.
Maloney Dilator	**Maloney dilator** is a bougie with a tapered end used in esophageal dilatation.
Hurst Dilator	**Hurst dilator** is a bougie filled with mercury for dilating the esophagus.
Savary-Gilliard Dilators	**Savary-Gilliard dilators** are polyvinyl dilators that have a channel for a guidewire.

Term	Definition
Rigiflex Dilators	**Rigiflex dilators** are pneumatic balloons use to dilate the lower esophageal sphincter.
French Units	**French units** are the measurement used to designate the size of an esophageal dilator. It reflects the circumference of the dilator.
Heater Probes	**Heater probes** are hollow aluminum cylinders with a heating coil to cause tissue coagulation.
Bipolar Probe	**Bipolar probe** is an electrode used in electrocoagulation in which the probe delivers the current and completes the circuit.
Monopolar Electrocoagulation	**Monopolar electrocoagulation** uses a single pole to produce coagulating current.
Electrosurgical Units	**Electrosurgical units** are instruments used to deliver electrocoagulation therapy.
Photocoagulation	**Photocoagulation** occurs at 60 C and causes tissue coagulation.
Photovaporization	**Photovaporization** occurs at 100 C and cuts or destroys tissue.
Ethamolin	**Ethamolin** is ethanolamine oleate, a sclerosing agent.
Sengstaken-Blakemore Tube	The **Sengstaken-Blakemore tube** is used in tamponade with a gastric and esophageal balloon.
Linton Tube	The **Linton tube** is used in tamponade but has no esophageal balloon.
Minnesota Tube	The **Minnesota tube** is used in tamponade. It has a gastric and esophageal balloon and also lumens to allow for both gastric and esophageal suction.
Billroth I	**Billroth I** is a surgical procedure for peptic ulcer disease in which the antrum of the stomach is removed with attachment of the duodenum to the remainder of the stomach.
Billroth II	**Billroth II** is a surgical procedure for peptic ulcer disease in which the upper duodenum and lower stomach are removed with the jejunum being attached to the remainder of the stomach.
Roux-En-Y	**Roux-en-Y** is a surgical procedure that creates a pouch in the proximal area of the stomach. The jejunum is attached to the pouch, and the duodenum is attached to the jejunum.
Esophageal Atresia	**Esophageal atresia** results at birth with the esophagus ending blindly, unattached to the stomach.
Nissen Fundoplication	**Nissen fundoplication** is used to strengthen the LES by wrapping the stomach around the lower esophagus and suturing it in place.

Patient Care Interventions

Emergency Interventions

Equipment Required in Gastroenterology Procedure Room for Emergency Resuscitation

Resuscitation equipment should be readily available in the gastroenterology procedure room so that a patient in distress can be quickly resuscitated. This equipment is in addition to monitoring equipment used during the procedure: pulse oximeters, ECG, automated sphygmomanometers, and capnography. Equipment required for emergency resuscitation includes:

- *Intravenous equipment*: Includes various IV and intraosseous bone marrow needles, syringes, tubing, and catheters.
- *Airway management equipment*: Suction equipment, catheters, airways, LMAA, laryngoscopes, endotracheal tubes, stylets, oxygen source, positive pressure equipment.
- *Reversal agents*: naloxone (Narcan®) and Romazicon (Flumazenil®).
- *Emergency medications*: Includes epinephrine, ephedrine, atropine, amiodarone, diphenhydramine, steroids, diazepam, midazolam, and lidocaine.
- *Defibrillator*

All equipment should be routinely checked to make sure it is operating condition. Medications should be rotated and expiration dates checked to ensure they are not outdated.

Investigating Source of Gastrointestinal Bleeding

Gastrointestinal bleeding can be minor, but it can also be life-threatening. The nurse helps to assess the patient, ascertaining vital signs, oxygenation and comfort. Appropriate measures must be instituted to offer support to the patient. The first course of action is medical stabilization. This may require central venous access, resuscitative efforts, or other invasive maneuvers. Once the patient is stabilized, searching for the source of bleeding becomes important so that corrective measures can be taken. Investigating for an upper gastrointestinal site may require placing a nasogastric tube, looking for blood. An endoscopy may be performed, depending on the medical stability of the patient. For lower gastrointestinal bleeds, an upper gastrointestinal source needs to be ruled out. A scan to follow tagged red blood cells may point to a source. A colonoscopy may be performed for visualization, if the patient can tolerate the procedure. Surgery is always a possibility in gastrointestinal bleeding.

Perforation of Gastrointestinal Tract

Perforation results in a hole in the gastrointestinal wall. This may be the result of trauma or underlying pathology. Although uncommon, endoscopic procedures can lead to perforations. Those at risk often have a predisposing factor, such as strictures or malignancies. Perforations in the upper gastrointestinal tract commonly present with pain. The location of the pain is related to the area of perforation. Gastric perforations are less common that esophageal perforations. Many perforations can be managed conservatively, although a surgical consult is needed. Patients who demonstrate complications, such as peritonitis, need immediate intervention. Perforations of the lower gastrointestinal tract are often asymptomatic. However, the symptoms can rapidly progress. Usually, these need surgical intervention.

Hypovolemic Shock

Shock is the state of a patient who cannot maintain his/her cardiovascular status. This may be due to blood or fluid loss or to factors that undermine the control of the circulatory system, such as sepsis. Hypovolemic shock results from a lack of body fluids to support the circulatory system. The body alters its circulatory priorities to favor central organs, such as the heart and the brain. This is done at the expense of other organ systems, such as the kidney. Patients are tachycardic and anxious. As the shock progresses, patients become hypotensive. Patients should be given appropriate volume support with fluids or other volume expanders. The feet should be elevated. Drugs to maintain perfusion may be used. Treating the underlying cause must be aggressively attempted, once the patient is stabilized.

Septic Shock

Septic shock can accompany bacteremia, leading to cardiovascular compromise. Any source of infection can lead to septic shock, including gastrointestinal infections. The patient may initially present with fever, chills, and borderline blood pressure. If untreated, this can progress to cardiovascular collapse, not unlike advanced hypovolemic shock. Treatment requires aggressive support of the patient, with fluids and blood pressure source. Treating for infection should begin immediately. Investigation of the source of infections should be addressed to implement appropriate corrective action. Some gastrointestinal procedures are associated with a rate of infections complications, such as ERCP or dilations. Most agree that antibiotics should be reserved for high risk patients, such as patients with a history of endocarditis.

Adverse Drug Reactions

Every medication has potential **side effects, or unwanted actions on the individual.** Being aware of these side effects can enable the clinician to anticipate adverse events. Actions to deal with adverse events can then be taken, as needed. In addition, cautious use and administration of any medication should always be pursued. Many individuals have allergies to medications, and some of those are unaware of their allergies. The clinician should always determine an allergic history, but should also be prepared for an unexpected allergic reaction. In addition, some individuals are allergic to latex, a ubiquitous substance in medical settings. There should always be a full array of emergency equipment available in the event that a patient needs to be resuscitated. For anaphylaxis, immediate treatment with epinephrine can minimize the adverse effects. Other supportive measures need to be implemented, as well.

Resuscitative Measures for Negative Response to Anesthesia

Negative responses to anesthesia vary according to the type of anesthetic agent administered, but can include:

- *Respiratory depression*: The dosage may need to be decreased. With opioid depression, naloxone may be administered; and with benzodiazepine depression, Romazicon (Flumazenil®). Supplementary oxygen and positive pressure ventilation may be required.
- *Airway obstruction*: Airway may require suctioning, jaw thrust, and administration of oxygen with a BVM to clear obstruction. Succinylcholine may be needed for laryngospasm, epinephrine for laryngeal edema, and albuterol and epinephrine for bronchospasm.
- *Hypotension/Bradycardia*: Treatment may include atropine, ephedrine, and/or phenylephrine.
- *Hypertension*: Treatment may include nitroglycerin and labetalol.

- *Malignant hyperthermia*: The anesthetic agent should be immediately discontinued although surgery may continue with different agents. The patient should be hyperventilated with 100% oxygen and Dantrolene 2.5 mg/kg and 1.2 mEq/kg of sodium bicarbonate administered IV through a central line or large bore IV. Ice packs are applied to groin, axillary, neck, wrists, and ankle, and iced lavage of stomach and rectum as needed to reduce temperature. Other treatments may include mannitol or furosemide, procainamide, calcium, and insulin.

Cardiac Arrest in Gastrointestinal Suite

Cardiovascular events are a potential side effect for patients undergoing procedures. Patients may be at risk from the actual procedure, increased anxiety or reactions to medications. For those at risk, EKG monitoring should be provided throughout the study. Emergency equipment should be available, and should be checked daily to assess function and completeness. If cardiac arrest occurs, CPR should be instituted. IV fluids and medications should be administered, and the airway should be secured. Outcomes are much more favorable for those who receive early action. Documentation of all events and actions is imperative.

Resuscitative Measures for Cardiac Arrest

Cardiopulmonary resuscitation for cardiac arrest:

- Immediate defibrillation (one shock) for VT/VF (shockable rhythms) according to protocol with manual defibrillator (preferred over AED) followed by CPR, beginning with compressions (30:2 compression to ventilation at the rate of 100-120 per minute at least 2 inches deep; 2-finger compressions, 1/3 chest depth for infants and children) for two minutes/5 cycles and repeat defibrillation. Non-shockable rhythms (PEA/asystole) do not respond to defibrillation.
- Obtain IV/IO access; begin PETCO2 if available.
- Administer epinephrine 1 mg every 3 to 5 minutes.
- Repeat cycles of 2 minutes CPR and defibrillation.
- If defibrillator is not readily available, CPR may begin first. Note if BVM is used, the break in compressions should not exceed 10 seconds. If an advanced airway/intubation is in place, ventilation should be at the rate of 8 to 10 per minutes, maintaining oxygen saturation ≥94% but <100% with ventilation between compressions.
- Adrenaline (IV 1 mg) and vasopressin (40 units) may be repeatedly administered with PEA, asystole, or VF and when two shocks have been unsuccessful.
- ETCO2 value should be 10-20 mm Hg if chest compressions are adequate, increasing to 35 to 45 mm Hg with return of spontaneous circulation (ROSC).

Respiratory Depression in the Gastroenterology Suite

Respiratory depression can result from some of the medications used during gastrointestinal procedures. Patients will demonstrate a decreased respiratory rate and a drop in oxygen saturation. Clinicians need to be cautious with the administration of medications. Certainly, titration rates should be slow, along with using the lowest effective dose. Modifications may be needed for the elderly or for those with underlying medical conditions. Increasing the oxygen provided to the patient is necessary and sometimes sufficient. Drugs that depress the respiratory system may have to be reversed with appropriate antagonists. With **respiratory arrest**, emergency measures should be instituted immediately, providing support for the airway and the cardiovascular system. CPR should be undertaken and appropriate medications should be administered.

Emergency Medications

Emergency medications include:

- *Romazicon (Flumazenil®):* Used to reverse the sedative effects of benzodiazepines (often used as sedation for medical procedures and surgery), such as alprazolam (Xanax®), midazolam (Versed®), clorazepate dipotassium (Tranxene®), and diazepam (Valium®). Romazicon does not, however, reverse respiratory depression. Romazicon is administered IV with a beginning dose of 0.2 mg over 30 seconds with repeat doses at one-minute intervals as needed. The second dose is 0.3 mg and the third and subsequent doses are 0.5 mg.
- *Atropine:* Used in emergency situations to treat asystole, ventricular fibrillation, and pulseless electrical activity, atropine increases heart rate. The dosage is usually 0.5-1 mg IV every 3-5 minutes to a maximum of 3 mg. Atropine is also an antidote for muscarinic poisoning caused by overdose of medications, such as bethanechol and cholinesterase inhibitors.
- *Naloxone (Narcan®):* Opioid antagonist rapidly reverses the effects of opioid overdose, such as from heroin or prescription opiates/opioids. The injectable form (IV, SQ, or IM) is more commonly used by medical personnel and is generally more effective than the nasal spray. Initial dosage is 0.4mg for adults/10 mcg/kg for children with dosages repeated at 2- to 3-minute intervals as needed. For postoperative opioid effects, initial dosage is 0.1 to 0.2 mg IV repeated at 2- to 3-minute intervals as needed.
- *Epinephrine:* Used to treat anaphylaxis and life-threatening allergic reactions. Administered SQ, IM, IV, or intracardiac, epinephrine is a bronchodilator and vasoconstrictor and restores cardiac function in those experiencing asystole. The usual SQ/IM dosage is 0.1% (1:1000) and IV/intracardiac dosage is 0.01% (1:10,000).

ASA Sedation Guidelines

The **ASA sedation guidelines** (2018) are intended for moderate (conscious) sedation used for procedures. Steps include:

1. *Pre-procedure evaluation:* Includes review of health records, physical examination and laboratory testing as indicated a few days or weeks prior to the procedure and re-evaluating the patient again before the procedure.
2. *Patient preparation:* Consult with specialist if indicated, ensure patient has informed consent and has been compliant with pre-procedure fasting.
3. *Patient monitoring:* LOC (every 5 minutes), oxygenation/ventilation (capnography, pulse oximetry), and hemodynamic with designated person responsible for monitoring and recording.
4. *Supplemental oxygen:* Use unless contraindicated by condition.
5. *Emergency interventions:* Resuscitative equipment and reversal agents for opioids (naloxone) and benzodiazepines (Romazicon) must be present with person trained in assessment and use available.
6. *Sedatives:* Combinations of drugs as appropriate may be used (benzodiazepines and dexmedetomidine) and analgesics (opioids).

7. Sedative (propofol, ketamine, etomidate) and analgesics (local anesthetics, NSAIDs, and opioids) intended for general anesthesia: Care must be consistent with that of general anesthesia and IV medications administered incrementally.
8. *Recovery care*: Monitor oxygenation, ventilation, and circulation every 5 to 15 minutes.

Assessing Patient's Airway Status Before, During, and After Anesthesia Administration

According to ASA guidelines, the patient's **airway status** must be continually evaluated and monitored:

- *Before anesthesia:* The patient's records should be reviewed for evidence of airway compromise, such as a history sleep apnea, COPD, asthma, or bronchospasm. The airway should be evaluated as part of the physical examination. Specialists should be consulted if indicated to provide guidance regarding sedation and maintenance of a patent airway.
- *During anesthesia*: The patient should receive supplemental oxygen unless specifically contraindicated by condition. The patient's capnography and pulse oximetry should be continuously monitored and the patient's general condition monitored for signs of respiratory distress/depression or hypoxemia.
- *After anesthesia*: The patient's oxygenation must be continually monitored until the patient is alert and responsive and no longer at risk for respiratory compromise. Ventilation and circulation should be assessed at 5- to 15-minute intervals or more often if indicated by condition.

Promoting Gastrointestinal Wellness

Nutrients

The **six basic nutrients** include carbohydrates, lipids, proteins, vitamins, minerals and water.

- *Carbohydrates* are immediately acted upon by the salivary enzyme, ptyalin, which produces disaccharides. These are further broken down in the small intestine into monosaccharides. These are absorbed and become part of the glucose metabolism that fuels the energy of each cell. Glucose is stored in the liver as glycogen.
- *Lipids* are hydrolyzed and once they enter the small intestine they are converted to triglycerides. In various forms, these are emulsified and absorbed in the small bowel.
- *Proteins* contain amino acids, some of which are necessary for continued health. After they are hydrolyzed in the stomach, they are further broken down for absorption by pancreatic enzymes. They are then absorbed.
- *Vitamins* are necessary for the health of the body. They include those that are fat soluble; Vitamins A, D, E, K. The balance of vitamins is water soluble.
- *Minerals* include substances such as calcium and phosphorus.
- *Water* is essential for cellular health, transport of nutrients and maintenance of body temperature.

Dietary Limitations

The following are various **dietary limitations**:

- **Dietary fiber** is important to maintain stool bulk and prevent constipation. Fiber can be provided through whole grains, fruits, vegetables or bran.
- For those suffering from diarrhea, a **low fiber** diet may be recommended.

- Those with celiac disease need to **avoid gluten-containing foods** such as wheat, rye, oats and barley. This is a difficult commitment, but patients should be encouraged because of the consequences, such as diarrhea and failure to thrive.
- **Avoidance of lactose** is needed for those who are lactose intolerant. This requires the avoidance of lactose-containing substances, such as milk. There are mild substitutes, as well as pills to that contain the missing enzyme, lactase.
- **Low protein diets** are required for those with severe liver or renal disease. Supplements may be added to prevent negative nitrogen balance.
- **Low fat diets** are often required to control gastrointestinal diseases that are accompanied by diarrhea of steatorrhea.
- **Low sodium diets** are often needed for patients with liver, renal or cardiac diseases.

Enteral Feedings

Enteral nutrition is provided for those who cannot adequately consume foods. This is useful for those who have a functioning gastrointestinal tract. It provides advantages of total parenteral nutrition because it is cheaper, is less invasive and is more tolerated. This form of nutrition is done through tubes accessing the gastrointestinal tract via the nose, the mouth or percutaneously. For long term access, a tube may be inserted surgically to the small bowel. The rate of feeding should be gradual, and then the concentration is gradually increased. This form of providing nutrition is less expensive and poses less risk than parenteral nutrition.

Common Problems

Aspiration is the most common **complication** in these patients. Other complications include vomiting, diarrhea, constipation, local necrosis from tube placement, and electrolyte imbalances. The nurse must monitor the patient carefully, as well as careful assessment of the tube placement with intermittent feedings. Patient education is important for appropriate administration and care of the access channel. Patients should be encouraged to exercise and to participate in normal activities. Patients should also be reminded that a more normal mode of feeding will be started as soon as possible.

TPN

Total parenteral nutrition provides for those who are unable to maintain their own nutritional balance independently. For this form of nutrition, an appropriate indwelling catheter should be placed. Peripheral nutrition can be offered for some individuals, such as those who need short term support. Total parenteral nutrition or TPN includes contains the essential nutrients that are obtained from a normal diet. The physician orders this on a daily basis. It requires careful calculation to meet the needs of the patient. Many hospitals have a dedicated team that addresses the needs of these patients. Complications may include sepsis, complications from central line placement, air embolism or thrombophlebitis.

Pain Management

Interventions for **pain management** includes:

- *Ambulation*: Helps to increase circulation, to reduce the risk of thromboembolism, and to promote autonomy. Patients should be encouraged to count steps and to regularly increase the count. A pedometer may be useful to help the patient monitor activity.

- *Medication*: The type of pain dictates the medical response. For example, gas pain may be relieved by antacids; heartburn associated with reflux, antacids; abdominal cramping associated with constipation, stool softeners and/or laxatives; abdominal cramping associated with diarrhea, antidiarrheals; and rectal pain associated with hemorrhoids/fissures/fistulas, topical lidocaine/steroid preparations. Patients may receive relief from discomfort with acetaminophen and/or NSAIDs. Opioids, which may cause constipation, are reserved for severe pain, such as post-surgical.
- *Positioning*: Changing positions may help to alleviate discomfort, but the type of positioning must be individualized depending on the type of discomfort and what works for the patient. If a patient has abdominal pain, for example, the patient may have some relief from elevating the knees or lying on the side with knees drawn up. If the patient has rectal pain, avoiding direct pressure to the rectal area may help to relieve discomfort.

HIPAA

Sensitive information is classified under **HIPAA** as protected health information (PHI), applies to all healthcare, including gastroenterology patients, and includes:

- Any information about an individual's past, present, or future health or condition (mental or physical).
- Provision of health care provided to the individual.
- Any information related to payment for healthcare services that can be used to identify the person.
- Identifying information: Name, address, Social Security number, birthdate) and any document or material that contains the identifying information (such as laboratory records).

Personal information can be shared with spouse, legal guardians, those with durable power of attorney for the patient, and those involved in care of the patient, such as physicians, without a specific release. HIPAA mandates privacy and security rules to ensure that health information and individual privacy is protected:

- *Privacy rule:* Protected information includes any information included in the medical record (electronic or paper), conversations between the doctor and other healthcare providers, billing information, and any other form of health information.
- *Security rule*: Any electronic health information must be secure and protected against threats, hazards, or non-permitted disclosure.

Obtaining Patient Consent Prior to Gastroenterology Procedures

Patients or their representatives must be asked directly for signed **informed consent** prior to gastroenterology procedures. Informed consent requires that the person be competent to give consent; has been apprised of risks, benefits, and alternatives; comprehends the information provided; and gives consent without coercion. Children <18, unless legally emancipated, lack the legal right to give consent for medical treatments except in those areas approved by law, such as for birth control, abortion, and HIV testing, and even these vary from one state to another, with some requiring parent notification. However, children must be included in discussions about treatment options in accordance to their age and level of understanding. While state laws vary in relation to informed consent, generally the provision of emergency treatment is permissible without informed consent if the patient is unable to consent. For example, an accident patient who is unconscious can be treated if next of kin is not available to give consent. Generally, dementia alone does not negate the need for informed consent although that may be provided by a legal representative.

Ethical Principles When Providing Patient Care

Key ethical principles to be aware of in providing patient care include:

- *Autonomy* is the ethical principle that the individual has the right to make decisions about his/her own care, based on informed consent and understanding of risks and benefits. Ensuring that a patient has provided informed consent supports autonomy.
- *Beneficence* is an ethical principle that involves performing actions that are for the purpose of benefitting another person.
- *Nonmaleficence* is an ethical principle that means healthcare workers should provide care in a manner that does not cause direct intentional harm to the patient (although sometimes an action or treatment may cause harm as a means to achieve good, such as chemotherapy).
- *Justice* is the ethical principle that relates to the distribution of the limited resources of healthcare benefits to the members of society. Distribution should be fair with all having equal access.
- *Veracity* refers to honesty and truth telling in all interactions with patients, families, and other healthcare providers.

Advance Directives

In accordance to Federal and state laws, gastroenterology patients have the right to self-determination in health care, including decisions about end of life care through **advance directives** such as living wills and the right to assign a surrogate person to make decisions through a **durable power of attorney**. Patients should routinely be questioned about an advanced directive as they may present at a healthcare organization without the document. Patients who have indicated they desire a **do-not-resuscitate** (DNR) order should not receive resuscitative treatments for terminal illness or conditions in which meaningful recovery cannot occur. Patients and families of those with terminal illnesses should be questioned as to whether the patients are Hospice patients. For those with DNR requests or those withdrawing life support, staff should provide the patient palliative rather than curative measures, such as pain control and/or oxygen, and emotional support to the patient and family. Religious traditions and beliefs about death should be treated with respect.

Potential Complications

Potential complications the gastroenterology patient may experience include:

- *Flare ups*: A sudden exacerbation of symptoms occurs with some gastrointestinal disorders, such as Crohn's disease. Flare-ups may be associated with patient's stopping or skipping doses of their medications, taking NSAIDs, taking antibiotics, or smoking. Flareups may also result from increased stress and certain foods (which may differ from one individual to another).
- *Drug reactions*: The adverse effects of many OTC and prescription drugs include GI problems, such as nausea, vomiting, and diarrhea. Many drugs of abuse adversely affect the GI system as well. For example, cocaine may cause intestinal infarction and opioids may cause severe constipation.

- *Drug interactions*: These interactions alter the effects of one or more drugs on the body when multiple drugs are taken, with the risk of interactions increasing with the number of drugs. Many drugs interact with grapefruit, inhibiting the metabolism of the drugs. Antacids may decrease the absorption of some drugs, such as digoxin and phenytoin, and increase absorption of others, such as pseudoephedrine. Sodium bicarbonate may decrease excretion of some drugs, such as amphetamines and aspirin.

Resources Available to the Gastroenterology Patient

Resources available to the gastroenterology patient include:

- *Palliative care*: Supportive are provided to help the patient manage symptoms, such as pain and nausea, in order to improve the patient's quality of life. Palliative care should be available at all levels of care and may be provided in the home as part of Home Health care and Hospice care.
- *Support groups*: Usually peer groups of those with similar problems, such as living with Crohn's disease, but led by a professional who can provide education and guidance. Often available through local hospital or medical groups at no cost to participants.
- *Financial assistance*: Some organizations provide care with a sliding scale, but assistance may be available through Medicaid (for healthcare) or Social Services, for assistance with living expenses and housing. In some cases, faith-based organization, such as the Salvation Army or Catholic Charities, may provide some financial assistance.
- *Social assistance*: Volunteer agencies, such as Friendly Visitors, and some senior citizen groups may provide companionship and some assistance, such as help in filing taxes and with transportation.

Medication Administration

Role of Gastroenterology Nurse in Medication Administration

Gastroenterology nurses administer medications, as well as educate patients about medications. Therefore, the nurse needs to understand and appreciate the different drugs used in the field of gastroenterology. This includes appropriate dosing, route of administration, side effects and drug interactions. The nurse needs to consider the patient's needs and limitations, taking into account the age of the patient, medical history, drug history and allergies. Careful attention must be paid to the patient's ability to understand and follow the instructions. Documentation is essential. This creates a record of therapy, patient response and untoward effects. This information can also be used to make changes in policy or to study medical interventions.

Safe Injection Practices for Medication Administration

Safe injection practice for medication administration should include methods to ensure safety for both the patient and the nurse:

- *Nurse*: Retractable needles and safety caps should be available on syringes. Used syringes and needles should never be recapped manually or bent but should be immediately disposed of in an appropriate secure hazardous waste receptacle.

- *Patient*: The dosage must be correct and the appropriate route (SQ, IM, IV) and injection technique selected for the medication and the syringe and needle should be the correct size for the volume and with the appropriate needle gauge and length. Multi-dose vials should be used for only one patient. <u>Multi-vials</u> should be kept away from immediate treatment areas if they are to be accessed at different times. When used, the vial septum must be disinfected with 70% isopropyl swab, air dried and, aseptic technique used when obtaining each dose, including a new sterile needle and syringe if multiple doses must be obtained for a patient.

Administration of Medications

Medications can be administered orally, topically or parenterally. Oral medications are commonly given by mouth, but may need to be administered through a nasogastric tube or other avenue. The nurse must consider the ability of the patient to swallow the substance safely and if the oral route is the most effective way to administer the medication. Medications given parenterally are introduced by the subcutaneous, intravenous or intramuscular route. Different medications require different routes of administration. In addition, some decisions about route of administration may depend on how quickly a response is needed to the medication.

Antacids

Antacids act to neutralize the acidic environment in the stomach. These substances usually contain aluminum hydroxide, aluminum phosphate, calcium carbonate or magnesium salts. These are short-acting solutions to deal with gastrointestinal complaints such as heartburn and dyspepsia. Caution needs to be taken about educating the patient about possible complications of these medications. Some of the components of these drugs can be absorbed, such as Magnesium or Calcium. Consideration of other medications and of other medical conditions may determine if an antacid is appropriate. Some antacids may interfere with the absorption of other medications. Antacids may precipitate other complications in individuals with other medical problems, such as heart failure or renal failure.

Antibiotics, Antiparasitics, Antiflatulents, and Antidiarrheals

Antibiotics are used in gastroenterology to treat a number of conditions. Nurses must be familiar with how these drugs work, how they are dosed and administered, how they interact with other drugs, and possible side effects. **Antiparasitic and antifungal agents** are used to treat the invasion by parasites or fungi. **Antidiarrheals** are prescribed to control diarrhea. These agents work by inhibiting gastrointestinal activity (opiates), reducing gastrointestinal secretions (Pepto-Bismol), and/or decreasing the amount of fluid in the waste products (Kaopectate). **Antiflatulents** are used to treat symptoms produced by gastrointestinal gas.

Anticholinergics, Cholinergics, and Antiemetics

Anticholinergics work on both acid secretion and motility. Anticholinergics block the receptors on parietal cells to inhibit acid production. These medications also block nerve impulses that are responsible for smooth muscle tone and contractions. This can result in slower gastric emptying. Side effects include dryness of mucosal surfaces, decreased bladder activity, constipation, and flushing. Anticholinergics should not be used in patients with certain underlying medical conditions. **Cholinergics** promote gastrointestinal motility and secretion. Because of some side effects, such as abdominal cramping, cholinergics have limited applications. **Antiemetics** are prescribed for the control of nausea and vomiting. In general, these substances work on the central nervous system to suppress the vomiting center of the brain.

Laxatives and Cathartics

Laxatives and cathartics can lead to bowel evacuation. These substances work in several ways, including increasing intralumenal pressure, stimulation, increasing the bulk of stool, lubrication or softening the stool. Laxatives are used to prepare the bowel for diagnostic studies, such as for colonoscopy. The mucosal surface must be visualized, which requires that the bowel be free of stool. Sometimes these substances promote the elimination of certain materials from the intestine. They are also used to soften the stool and to treat constipation.

Medications for Ulcers

Medications used to treat ulcer disease work by reducing the effects of gastric acid or reducing the gastric acid itself.

- **H2 blockers or histamine 2 blockers** exert their effect on the gastric parietal cell to inhibit acid secretion. Adverse effects may include diarrhea, dizziness or blood dyscrasias.
- **Sucralfate** acts on duodenal ulcers as a buffer to the effects of gastric acid by covering the mucosal area. The most common adverse outcome is constipation.
- **Prostaglandins** are prescribed to prevent ulcer formation and to minimize any mucosal disturbances. Side effects include diarrhea and abdominal pain.
- **Proton pump inhibitors** act to interfere with the formation of gastric acid. People may develop abdominal pain, constipation, diarrhea, vomiting or headaches.

Medications for Inflammatory Diseases

Corticosteroids are useful in treating inflammatory disorders of the gastrointestinal tract, such as inflammatory bowel disease. Prolonged use can lead to certain complications, such as hypertension or osteoporosis. **Immune modulating agents** are used to attempt to reduce the exposure to prolonged steroids in patients with inflammatory bowel. These agents have some side effects that need careful monitoring, such as bone marrow suppression. Both of the above medications can impede an individual's ability to fight off infections. It is important for these patients to be up-to-date on all immunizations.

Medications to Treat Pain and Anesthetize Patients

Narcotic analgesics are used in gastroenterology to treat pain and to premedicate individuals. These agents can mask symptoms, however, so their use requires caution. **Sedatives and antianxiety agents** are most often used to produce conscious sedation in patients undergoing certain endoscopic procedures. Administration of these agents requires that the patient be carefully monitored through the procedure and after to be sure that vital signs and oxygenation are stable. Patients are at risk of respiratory depression, so equipment for resuscitation must be readily available. **Reversal agents** should also be available. These substances can reverse some of the effects of narcotics or sedatives.

Biologics

Biologics are drugs produced from natural sources, such as from cells derived from animals, microorganisms, and plants, or through DNA biotechnology. Biologics include monoclonal antibodies, cytokines, enzymes, growth factors, and immunomodulators. Biologics that block

- 78 -

inflammatory reactions, such as adalimumab, golimumab, infliximab, certolizumab, and natalizumab, are used to treat Crohn's disease and ulcerative colitis, usually if those conditions have not responded to more traditional treatments. These drugs help to bring about and sustain remission. Biologics also have a role in treatment of *Clostridium difficile* infection and eosinophilic esophagitis. Biologics are administered IV or SQ and cannot be taken orally. Adverse effects associated with biologics include local irritation, immunosuppression and increased risk of infection, and increased risk of lymphoma, joint pain and swelling, liver disease, and lupus-like reaction. Biologics may have reduced effectiveness if stopped and restarted because the patient may develop antibodies against the drug.

Probiotics

Probiotics are dietary supplements comprised of bacteria (such as lactobacilli and bifidobacteria) and yeast (*Saccharomyces boulardii*). Probiotics contain microorganisms that are part of the normal flora of the intestines and can help to restore the balance of microorganisms and improve the metabolism of foods and absorption of nutrients. Probiotics may also reduce colonization of pathogenic organisms. Probiotics that contain *Saccharomyces boulardii* also may help to reduce toxins produced by *Clostridium difficile.* Generally, probiotics are well-tolerated but they may cause some abdominal distention and cramping, especially with first taken. Patients who are severely immunocompromised and taking long-term broad- spectrum antibiotics have developed sepsis, so probiotics should be used with care in these patients. As with naturally-occurring bacteria and fungi, those in probiotics can be destroyed by antibiotics and fungicides, so probiotics should not be taken within two hours of these types of drugs.

Sedation Requirements for Different Procedures

The American Society of Anesthesiologists defines different **levels of anesthesiology** that can be used for gastroenterology procedures. These classifications are:

- *Minimal sedation*: patients respond normally to commands.
- *Moderate sedation*: also known as conscious sedation-state in which patients can respond to verbal stimuli, sometimes requiring stimulation
- *Deep sedation*: patients cannot be readily aroused without stimuli.
- *General anesthesia*: patients demonstrate loss of consciousness without arousability. Ventilatory capacity must be monitored carefully.

Each case is individual and requires careful evaluation and monitoring by the nurse. In general, the moderate sedation level or conscious sedation is usually adequate for endoscopic procedures.

Responsibilities of the Gastroenterology Nurse for Conscious Sedation

The registered nurse must assess the patient for the ability to communicate and cooperate, underlying medial conditions, pre-determined level of comfort, and ability to comply with pre-procedural requirements. The nurse must also ascertain that laboratory studies are within normal limits, that the consent form is signed, that the patient has followed pre-procedural orders and that the patient is aware of the procedure and its complications. Before and during the procedure, the nurse must be certain of the stability of vital signs, such as blood pressure, pulse, oxygen saturation and respiratory rate. These also need to be monitored following the procedure. Useful but not required are cardiac monitoring or automatic blood pressure monitoring. Sometimes, a second nurse is required for those patients with special needs, such as children. Documentation is very important. This should be done every 5 minutes during the period of anesthesia administration,

- 79 -

then every 15 minutes after sedation. Also, procedures, adverse reactions and therapies must be noted.

Choosing an Intravenous Site

Much of the choice rests with what is to be administered and for how long. Certainly, a **venous site must be chosen**. Arteries, unlike venous sites, pulsate. Avoid arteries for IV infusion. Saline or heparin locks can be placed to provide access without the administration of continuous IV fluids. With an IV infusion, a vein is accessed for the puncture. If a replacement is needed, it should be done proximally to the preceding site. For adults, lower extremity access should be avoided because those areas may be prone to thrombophlebitis. The lower extremity is acceptable for younger patients; infants may even be accessed via scalp veins. Documentation of substances given through the intravenous line must be ongoing.

Introducing an Intravenous Line

The area to be used should be appropriately disinfected. A tourniquet placed proximal to the access site increases the venous pressure so that a vein can be accessed. Gentle palpation across the targeted site can indicate venous tissue. Using the fingers, the vessel can be anchored above and below with the fingers to accommodate the needle. With appropriate insertion, there is a blood return. Once the needle has entered the vein, the plastic catheter can be gently advanced. It is then anchored with tape and antiseptic ointment should be applied. The site can then be hooked to IV tubing, or a special stop cock can be applied for a heparin lock. For removal, after clamping the IV, the catheter is removed. Appropriate pressure and dressing should be applied.

Complications Associated with Intravenous Therapy

Intravenous therapy is associated with some **complications**. Since the catheter penetrates the skin, there is an increased risk of infection. Careful attention needs to be paid to infection control. For long term in-dwelling access, there should be a schedule outlined for changes to reduce the risk of infection. Changing the intravenous equipment may reduce the chance of infections. If an infection is questioned, cultures should be taken. Other possible complications include: hematomas, phlebitis, air embolism, catheter embolism and fluid overload. Personnel are also at risk of needlesticks or other exposures to bodily fluids, which may lead to contamination and infection.

Methods of Giving Intravenous Medication

Giving medication intravenously requires that the nurse check the appropriateness of the order, the history of the patient, the compatibility of the medication, and the expiration date of the medicine. The patient's identity must be ascertained prior to giving the dose.

The **methods of administration** can include:

- *Continuous infusion*, in which the medicine is diluted in a liquid and dripped into the patient over a period of time.
- *Piggyback method*, in which the medication is hooked to the intravenous line in a separate container and given over a short period of time.
- *Intermittent infusion*, in which the intravenous access is maintained via a heparin lock for medications to be given at regular intervals.
- *IV bolus*, in which a discrete amount of medication is pushed over a short time by using an existing access.

Administering Blood Products

Whole blood can be administered, but fractionated components are preferred. Whole blood can be separated into red cells, platelets, plasma, and clotting factors.

- **Packed red blood cells** contain only erythrocytes and are administered for anemia.
- **Platelets** are given to those with very low platelets to circumvent bleeding.
- **Plasma** is the fluid part of the blood that contains clotting factors without platelets. This is used to treat clotting disorders.
- **Cryoprecipitates** are given to people with blood clotting factor deficiencies.

In administering blood, a filter is used to remove debris found in whole blood and packed cells. The right product must go into the right patient, so careful inspection and documentation is essential. The patient must also be monitored for adverse effects.

Adverse Reactions to Blood Products

Adverse reactions to blood products can occur. These include:

- *Volume overload*, in which the volume load overcomes the ability of heart to pump it. This leads to pulmonary edema.
- *Bacterial reactions* from contaminated blood, manifesting as fever, chills and pain.
- *Allergic reactions* from exposure to substances in the blood that cause an allergic response
- *Hemolytic reactions* from being exposed to incompatible blood.
- *Subsequent infections* from virus contaminated blood.

Once an adverse reaction is noted, the transfusion should be stopped immediately. After stabilizing the patient, the blood should be returned to the blood bank with documentation of the reaction.

Important Terms

Term	Definition
Hemolysis	**Hemolysis** is the lysis of red blood cells.
Vascular Access Devices	**Vascular access devices** are for long term use. They include central venous line devices and indwelling infusion ports.
Osmosis	**Osmosis** is the process by which solvents pass through a selectively permeable membrane.
PCA	**PCA** or **patient-controlled analgesic** devices are patient controlled intravenous access devices for the delivery of pain medication.
Infiltration	**Infiltration** occurs when substances from the inserted intravenous line leak into surrounding tissue.
Leukocyte-Poor Blood	**Leukocyte-poor blood** is blood used for prospective transplant patients because it reduces the likelihood of sensitization to tissue antigens.
Phlebitis	**Phlebitis** is an inflammation of the vein, which can occur as a complication of intravenous therapy.
Perforation	**Perforation** is an opening through the wall of the gastrointestinal tract.
Hematochezia	**Hematochezia** occurs when the individual has bloody stools.
Melena	**Melena** occurs when the individual produces odiferous, tarry stools.
Hematemesis	**Hematemesis** is vomiting blood.
Boerhaave's Syndrome	**Boerhaave's syndrome** results in a perforation that occurs spontaneously, usually associated with vomiting.
Bacteremia	**Bacteremia** is the presence of bacterial organisms in the blood.
Anaphylaxis	**Anaphylaxis** is a severe allergic reaction that results in cardiovascular collapse and possibly death.
Cheyne-Stokes Respirations	**Cheyne-Stokes respirations** are periods of increased respirations interspersed with periods of decreased respirations.
Vasovagal Syncope	**Vasovagal syncope** is a transient loss of consciousness due to a neurologic and cardiovascular response to fear or pain.
Aspiration	**Aspiration** is the inappropriate introduction of substances to the respiratory system.
Positive Nitrogen Balance	**Positive nitrogen balance** results when protein synthesis exceeds protein degradation.
Negative Nitrogen Balance	**Negative nitrogen balance** results when protein degradation exceeds protein intake.
Enteral Nutrition	**Enteral nutrition** is provided for those who cannot eat but who have functioning bowels.
Percutaneous Endoscopic Gastrostomy	**Percutaneous endoscopic gastrostomy** requires insertion of a gastrostomy feeding tube via the endoscope.
Percutaneous Endoscopic Jejunostomy	**Percutaneous endoscopic jejunostomy** requires insertion of a jejunostomy feeding tube via endoscopy.
Total Parenteral Nutrition	**Total parenteral nutrition** or **TPN** is nutritional supplementation for the patient with gastrointestinal dysfunction.
Amino Acids	**Amino acids** are the combined to form proteins.
Minerals	**Minerals** are nutrients that are inorganic.
Vitamins	**Vitamins** are nutrients that are organic.

Term	Definition
Peptavlon	**Peptavlon** is pentagastrin, a drug used that causes an increase in gastric acid secretion.
Chymex	**Chymex** is bentiromide, which helps evaluate the exocrine function of the pancreas.
Tensilon	**Tensilon** is edrophonium chloride, used to stimulate esophageal spasm.
Secretin	**Secretin** can be administered to investigate the exocrine function of the pancreas.
Glucagon	**Glucagon**, which decreases motility, may be used for different procedures.
Kinevac	**Kinevac** is cholecystokinin and is used to cause the gallbladder to contract.
Chenix	**Chenix** or chenodeoxycholic acid is used to dissolve cholesterol gallstones.
Actigall	**Actigall** or ursodeoxycholic acid is used to dissolve cholesterol gallstones.
Monooctanoin	**Monooctanoin** is used to dissolve cholesterol gallstones.
Meperidine	**Meperidine** or Demerol is a narcotic analgesic that is especially useful in biliary or pancreatic diseases.
Fentanyl	**Fentanyl** or Sublimaze is a narcotic analgesic associated with less nausea and vomiting.
Narcan	**Narcan** or naloxone is used to reverse sedation and respiratory depression caused by opioids.
Romazicon	**Romazicon** or flumazenil can reverse the sedation of benzodiazepines.
Sclerosing Agents	**Sclerosing agents** are used to thrombose and fibrose varices.
Isordil	**Isordil** is used to treat esophageal spasm.
Procardia	**Procardia** or nifedipine is a calcium channel blocker used to relax the LES.

Environment Safety, Infection Prevention and Control

Standard Infection Control

Infection Control

<u>Purpose</u>

The risk of infection must be controlled effectively in gastroenterology. Procedures and treatments increase a patient's risk of infection. It is important that all equipment be appropriately cleaned, sterilized or disinfected according to standards. Earl Spaulding classified devices in the endoscopy suite by level of risk of infection to patients.

- Equipment that is used with the intent to disturb the mucosal surface of the gastrointestinal tract is deemed critical and requires sterilization.
- Instruments that have contact with skin and mucous membranes are considered semicritical and require high-level disinfection.
- Noncritical objects come in contact with skin only and pose a reduced risk of infection. They require intermediate or low-level disinfection.

<u>Different Levels of Infection</u>

Appropriate measures must be taken to keep equipment that comes into contact with patients as clean as possible. There are different demands for preparing different instruments before they are used on patients. Some instruments require **sterilization**, the process of getting rid of all microorganisms. This is accomplished by different methods, such as autoclave (steamed heat), dry heat, use of ethylene oxide at low temperatures, and use of certain disinfectants. The process of **disinfection** can be carried out at several levels.

- *High level* has the most killing potential, destroying mycobacteria, viruses, fungi and vegetative bacteria.
- To achieve *intermediate-level,* the process must lead to inactivating M. tuberculosis, vegetative bacteria, most viruses, and most fungi.
- *Low-level* kills most organisms but does not work against M. tuberculosis.

Standard PPE During Patient Procedures

According to CMS guidelines, patient procedures, such as endoscopic examinations, must be carried out under the same standards as surgical operations in a sterile operating/procedure room although most endoscopic procedures, such as a colonoscopy, have been traditionally considered non-sterile. **Personal protective equipment (PPE)** for sterile environments includes gloves, impervious gown, head and foot coverings, and face mask and face or eye shields. The same PPE is utilized in endoscope reprocessing areas, which should be separate from the procedure room. Some organizations (AORN, AAMI) also require application of clean scrubs provided by the workplace. Handwashing is especially important and should be carried out before gloves are applied and after removal. PPE should be removed and discarded appropriately after a procedure and before leaving the procedure room. For care after the procedure, such as in the recovery area, PPE should be utilized according to risk, but usually includes gown and gloves.

Appropriate Care for Thermal Burns, Chemical Spills, and Radiation

Appropriate care for these issues on the gastroenterology unit include:

- *Thermal burns:* Bipolar probes/electrocautery are used to seal vessels with heat but may cause thermal injury and even perforations of the colon, which require surgical repair. Post-polypectomy electrocoagulation syndrome, (transmural burn but without perforation), which mimics the symptoms of perforations but heals with conservative treatment, may also occur. CT can differentiate the two conditions.
- *Chemical spills:* Spills may occur in any setting and may be small (up to 300 mL), medium (up to 5L), and large (greater than 5L) and may require neutralization and/or absorption with a spill kit. Large spills may require outside assistance. Some spills require alerts and evacuation while others require only restriction from the area of the spill. Material Data Safety Sheets should be consulted for appropriate response.
- *Radiation:* Patients are often exposed to high levels of ionizing radiation, especially with the increased use of computed tomography and x-rays. Exposure should be limited as much as possible and adequate shielding provided during imaging.

"Time-Out" Prior to Procedure Initiation

The pre-surgical/procedural **time-out** is part of the Joint Commission's Universal Protocol for preventing surgical/procedural errors. The time-out procedure, which should follow a standard format, follows completion of pre-procedure verification and marking of the procedure site (if appropriate) and includes:

- A designated team member initiates the time-out before beginning an invasive procedure/incision.
- All team members who will participate in the procedure must be present and all must communicate during the time-out.
- The entire team must agree that they have the correct patient and the correct site and must agree on the procedure that is scheduled.
- If a patient is scheduled for more than one procedure, a time-out must be called prior to the beginning of all subsequent procedures.
- If those performing the procedure change during the procedure, for example if another physician takes over, another time-out must be called.
- Each time-out must be documented.

Equipment Reprocessing

Reprocessing of Accessory Equipment

Forceps need high level sterilization. These devices need both manual cleaning and manual sterilization. Reprocessing the **water bottle** requires cleaning, lubricating and sterilizing/disinfecting the water bottle. The water bottle consists of the water container, the cap and the tubing that attaches the bottle to the flexible endoscope. On a daily basis, the water bottle must be manually cleansed and sterilized/disinfected according to the manufacturers' specifications. The bottle must be stored dry with no residual liquid or moisture remaining. This will reduce the likelihood of bacterial colonization. Sterile water must be used for all endoscopic procedures. During ERCPs, a reprocessed water bottle must be used for each procedure. ERCPs have a risk of infections.

Bioburden

Bioburden refers to viable microorganisms that are present on an item, such as an endoscope, before sterilization or present in a liquid. Bioburden is especially a concern in gastroenterology because many nosocomial infections have been endoscopy-associated because of improper reprocessing and disinfection. Bioburden is described in terms of colony-forming units per milliliter (CFU/mL) or total viable count (TVC) of bacteria and fungi and is most often used in reference to bioburden testing (microbial limit testing) that is carried out on medical supplies and products. However, bioburden may also be used to describe the number of organisms (load and diversity) present in a wound or infection, helping to determine the choice of antibiotic or other treatment; and bioburden is used to describe environmental contamination. For example, a high level of *Clostridium difficile* bioburden increases the risk of outbreak, and control measures focus on decreasing the bioburden.

Sterilization and High Level Disinfection

Spaulding Classification for Surface Sterilization and Disinfection

Earle H. Spaulding (1957) devised a classification scheme for disinfection and sterilization of patient care equipment and supplies:

- *Critical items* are those that come in contact with sterile tissue and/or the vascular system, including surgical instruments, needles, and angiocaths. These items require sterilization (steam heat, ethylene oxide gas, chemical sterilants) because they carry a high risk of infection.
- *Semi-critical items* include those that come in contact with mucous membranes and non-intact skin, including anesthesia equipment, respiratory equipment, endocavitary probes, and scopes. These items require high-level disinfection (pasteurization, chemical sterilants, such as >2% glutaraldehyde) to remove all organisms although a small number of spores may remain.
- *Noncritical items* are those that come in contact with intact skin only and have no contact with mucous membranes, including blood pressure cuffs, urinals, bedpans, and assistive devices. Noncritical items include both those items that come in contact with the patient and with environmental surfaces. These items require intermediate-level (does not destroy spores) to low-level disinfectant (does not destroy spores or mycobacteria).

Cleaning the Endoscope

When the endoscope is removed from the patient, the surface of the instrument should be wiped with a cloth freshly prepared with enzyme detergent solution. The cloth should then be disposed of or sterilized/disinfected. The distal end of the endoscope should be placed into a container of detergent solution. The solution should be suctioned through the biopsy/suction channel until it appears visibly clear. The detergent suction should be alternated with air suction. The endoscope should then be flushed out or blown out as directed by the manufacturer. At this point, the endoscope should be detached from the light source and the suction pump. If video equipment is used, affix the protective video cap. The endoscope should be inspected for leaks and other damage. The instrument and appropriate parts should be brushed while in the detergent solution. The endoscope should be placed in the container and covered, to prevent exposure/spillage.

The **endoscope** needs high level disinfection. The instrument must be submerged in the disinfectant for 20 minutes. After the appropriate time, time endoscope channels need to be flushed with air, then thoroughly rinsed. Channels should be flushed with air and then rinsed with alcohol, then flushed with air again. The endoscope should be totally free of chemicals to avoid exposing a future patient to them. The most commonly used disinfectant for this purpose is glutaraldehyde. Before storage the endoscope should be thoroughly dry to reduce bacterial colonization. The endoscope should be stored vertically. There are some automated reprocessors available. Thorough pre-cleaning is still necessary, however. In addition, determining if the automatic reprocessor provides sufficient cleaning for some scopes, such as the ERCP scope, must be ascertained.

HDL Disinfection of Endoscopes

All endoscopes need to undergo **high disinfection level (HDL) disinfection**. Choosing which chemicals depends on manufacturing guidelines in relation to the endoscope. Personnel should be familiar with SDS/safety data sheets for all of the chemicals. Disposal of containers and chemicals must be done according to recommendations by the manufacturer. Spill kits need to be available at all times. Appropriate personal protective equipment must be worn by staff. These recommendations are given by the manufacturer. An eyewash station must be accessible. All of the internal channels need to have a flow of the disinfectant. The external surfaces must come in contact with the chemicals. A record of all reprocessing should be kept in case of future problems with contamination. Heating and air conditioning vents should be evaluated regularly.

Sterilization/Disinfection with Single Use Devices Versus Reusable Devices

Single-use devices (suction catheters, stylets, ETTs) are those intended to be discarded as hazardous waste immediately after a single use. These devices typically come in sealed sterile packs and require no further sterilization or disinfection. Some new single-use endoscopes, for example, are disposable and cannot be reprocessed so that the risk of cross-contamination is eliminated. However, some devices are **reusable** and some single-use devices may legally be reprocessed for additional use. According to the FDA, reprocessing should be done in most circumstances by third-party reprocessors because reprocessing must meet stringent industry standards. Cleaning/reprocessing activities must be done in a separate reprocessing area from the procedure room. Personnel must be thoroughly trained, and reprocessing should begin immediately after use. The device should be disassembled and parts cleaned with an enzymatic detergent, being sure to repeatedly flush and brush all channels to remove all organic material. All brushes or devices used for cleaning should be disposable or disinfected/sterilized between use. Ultrasonic cleaning may be used to clean areas that are hard to clean manually. After manual cleaning, devices should receive high-level disinfection by immersion or sterilization as appropriate.

Minimal Effective Concentration of Disinfection Solutions

The **minimal effective concentration** of disinfection solutions is the lowest concentration that is effective in destroying pathogenic organisms and/or spores within a specified duration of time. The concentration varies according to the type of disinfectant and whether it is used for high-level or low-level disinfection. Additionally, different concentrations may be needed for different organisms and different durations of exposure. Examples include:

- *Glutaraldehyde 2%:* Contains 1.0% to 1.5% active ingredient, sufficient to destroy pathogens.
- *Alcohol*: Low-level disinfection only, does not destroy spores or penetrate organic material. Ethyl alcohol at 60-80% is viricidal for lipophilic viruses and some hydrophilic viruses, 95% is effective for *M. tuberculosis*, 70% for many bacteria.

- *Hypochlorites*: 5.25% to 6.15% (equal to 52,500 to 61,500 ppm); 1000 ppm needed for *M. tuberculosis,* but 100 ppm needed for many bacteria and spores and 200 ppm for viruses. 1:10 dilution provides 5250-6150 ppm. Common dilutions for disinfection include 1:10 to 1:100.
- *Formaldehyde*: Sold as formalin at 37% formaldehyde and is effective against bacteria, viruses, fungi, spores, and *M. tuberculosis,* but formaldehyde is a carcinogen so exposure and use are limited.

Electrical, Laser, Radiation, and Chemical Safety

Electrical Safety Practices

Electrical safety must be respected. All connections need to be checked regularly, including electrical outlets. Care should be used with flammable materials. Both manufacturers' instructions concerning equipment and institutional policies should be followed. Appropriate fire safety precautions should be taken, including regular checks of safety equipment. All equipment should be checked to be certain of normal functioning. Precautions need to be taken for patients with allergies, such as to latex, need to be considered. Appropriate precautions need to be taken for patients and personnel alike. Preventive measures need to be instituted to reduce accidental injuries.

Safety Measures When Using Electrocautery Devices

Electrocautery uses high-radio-frequency electrical current to cut or coagulate areas in the gastrointestinal tract. The lowest setting possible should be used to accomplish the goals. When not in use, the device should be turned off or set to standby mode. The equipment should be checked regularly by appropriate personnel so that it is in good working order. Prior to use in the endoscopy suite, check the integrity of the instrument. Bipolar models may be safer since the current returns through the instrument and not the patient. Monopolar models require the appropriate placement of dispersive electrodes or grounding pads for the respective patient. Patients with an implantable defibrillator should have it turned off for the procedure. For patients with pacemakers, special care needs to be taken. The appropriate action should be checked with the patient's cardiologist, and all manufacturing guidelines should be followed.

Laser Safety

Lasers are used for coagulation and to vaporize tissue. Use of laser equipment can cause fire, skin or eye damage and irritation of the respiratory tract for everyone in the room. Only necessary personnel should be in the room and a warning sign on the door should advise that a laser is in use. Appropriate eye protection should be worn by patients and personnel to protect vision. When not in use, the laser should remain in standby mode. To reduce respiratory exposure, employ smoke evacuators or masks. Move combustible materials away from possible laser contact.

Safety of Glutaraldehyde in Endoscopy Suites

For all chemicals: follow label instructions, be familiar with the safety data sheets on these chemicals, and be aware of the spill containment procedure. **Glutaraldehyde** is soluble in water and which can vaporize easily. These properties result in the chemical causing irritation of the eyes and mucous membranes. To minimize exposure, personnel handling glutaraldehyde should wear rubber gloves, goggles, face shield/mask, and an impervious gown. Have access to an eye wash and other washing facilities to flush eyes or wash skin. Wash all personal protective equipment before it is used again. Use of glutaraldehyde should be restricted to areas with appropriate ventilation to reduce respiratory exposure. Storage requires a cool, dry location. The chemical should be stored in a covered container.

Minimizing Radiation Exposure

The use of X-rays and fluoroscopy in the diagnosis of gastrointestinal diseases is very useful. Radiation exposure can be harmful, so minimizing exposure is very important. Those in the endoscopy suite are exposed to **radiation** in three ways: primary, secondary and leakage from the equipment.

- *Primary exposure* occurs to the individual being studied. The radiation source is directed at the area to be investigated.
- *Secondary radiation* occurs when primary radiation scatters or bounces off surfaces. This is the main exposure for the staff in the room.

Staff members should limit their time in the exam room and allow the greatest possible distance from the source of radiation. Individuals should wear protective gear including a lead apron, thyroid shield, lead glasses, and radioprotective gloves. Shields can be erected around the examination table to reduce exposures. All members with radiation exposure need to wear monitoring equipment to track exposure levels.

Safe Handling of Body Piercings

Body piercing jewelry should be removed prior to gastroenterology procedures because those on the tongue, lip or nose may interfere with visualization of the airway and may become dislodged and aspirated. Body piercings may conduct electricity, causing burns, if electrocautery is utilized. Piercings may also interfere with imaging, causing artifacts, and cause burns or punctures if left in place during an MRI. Removal procedures vary:

- Nose studs: Apply gentle pressure and pull straight out.
- Nose screws with curved circle at the end: Slowly twist out.
- Barbell-type (used on face, lips, genitals, nipples, and navel): Unscrew end bead, counter-clockwise.
- Enclosed ring (used on face lips, genitals, nipples, and navel): Apply pressure inside the ring to force ends apart.
- Labret stems: Unscrew end backpiece, counterclockwise.

Some patients will want the tract maintained. In such cases, sutures or small catheters may be fed through the tract or non-metallic retainers placed if they do not interfere with the procedure or increase risk to the patient.

Proper Body Mechanics/Ergonomics and Prevention of Repetitive Strain Injuries

Proper **body mechanics/ergonomics** and prevention of repetitive strain injury include:

- Avoid bending at the waist to lift or reach for items. Stoop down with the knees bent.
- Avoid stretching overhead to reach for items on high shelves or out of reach. Use a step stool or grip tool with extension.
- Avoid pushing or pulling with the arms. Use the whole body to relieve strain on the arms and back.

- Avoid reaching, bending, or twisting to lift. Stand close to the person or item to be lifted, bend knees and hips, and use the muscles in the legs to support weight rather than the back or arms.
- Avoid lifting. Use lift devices rather than manually lifting heavy items and patients.
- Avoid prolonged periods of repetitive activity, such as keyboarding or stocking materials and take not of numbness and tingling or discomfort (warning signs). Take frequent short breaks.

Environmental Safety, Infection Prevention and Control

Multidrug Resistance

VRE and MDRO

Vancomycin *resistant enterococci* (VRE) and multi-drug resistant organisms (MDR0), such as multi-drug resistant *enterococci,* have become severe cause for concern. VRE was first identified in the United States in 1989, but by 2004 it was the cause of one-third of all hospital-acquired infections in intensive care units, related to the use of vancomycin. There are several phenotypes, but 2 types are most common in the United States: VanA (resistant to vancomycin and teicoplanin) and Van B (resistant to just van VRE) infections are treatable by other antibiotics, but MDRO infections are increasingly resistant to 2 or more antibiotics, including vancomycin. Restriction of vancomycin use alone has not proven successful in controlling development of VRE or MDRO because other antibiotics, such as clindamycin, cephalosporin, aztreonam, ciprofloxacin, aminoglycoside, and metronidazole are implicated. Prior antibiotic use is present in almost all patients with MDRO. Other risk factors include prolonged hospitalization and intraabdominal surgery.

CRE

Carbapenem-resistant Enterobacteriaceae (CRE), such as *Klebsiella* sp. and *Escherichia coli*, are normally found in the human intestinal system but are difficult to treat because of their resistance to almost all (and in some cases, all) antibiotics, resulting in death in up to half of those with bloodstream infections. Enzymes that break down both carbapenems (a usual target for antibiotics) and antibiotics, rendering them ineffective, include:

- *Klebsiella pneumoniae* carbapenemase (KPC): Most common in US.
- New Delhi Metallo-beta-lactamase (NDM-1): Associated with treatment in Pakistan or India.
- Verona Integron-Mediated Metallo-beta-lactamase (VIM): Found in *Pseudomonas.*
- Imipenemase metallo-beta lactamase (IMP).

Infections are associated with patients who have exposure to healthcare settings, such as hospitals and long-term care facilities; invasive medical devices, such as mechanical ventilators and catheters; and long-term antibiotic treatment. CRE is easily transmitted person-to-person, especially with contact with fecal material or open wounds. Some patients may be colonized but asymptomatic. CRE may be transmitted with inadequately sterilized endoscopes.

Patient Education Regarding Crohn's Disease

Important elements of patient education for patients with **Crohn's disease** (regional ileitis) includes:

- Patients need to know the usual signs and symptoms and progression of the disease (diarrhea, anemia, abdominal pain, nausea and vomiting, malabsorption, fever, night sweats, and perirectal abscess/fistula) as well as common treatments (steroids, antibiotics, immunomodulatory agents, antidiarrheals, aminosalicylates, tumor necrosis factor antagonists and enteral feedings or TPN).
- Patients should understand possible adverse effects associated with treatment and be alert for complications.
- Patients should be aware of the pattern of flareups and remission that is common to Crohn's disease and other problems that may occur, such as aphthous stomatitis, inflammation of the joints and eyes and anal fissures, fistulas, and ulcerations.
- Patients must be aware of lifestyle changes that may help to reduce symptoms and flareups, such as avoiding NSAIDS, exercising regularly, and stopping smoking. Patients should be aware of increased risk of colon cancer.

Patient Education Regarding *C. Diff,* VRE, and CRE

Clostridium difficile (C.diff), **vancomycin-resistant enterococci (VRE),** and **Carbapenem-resistant Enterobacteriaceae (CRE)** result in healthcare associated infections. Important elements of patient education include:

- *Cause of the infection*: Infections occur in those exposed to healthcare settings, invasive medical devices, and/or long-term or repeated antibiotic therapy. C.diff is caused associated with clindamycin and cephalosporins although all antibiotics have been implicated. VRE and CRE may result from almost all antibiotics.
- *Signs and symptoms*: C.diff results in severe diarrhea but may progress to sepsis. Both CRE and VRE may result in many different types of life-threatening infections (pneumonia, sepsis, UTI, wound infection).
- *Transmission*: Some patients infected with these organisms are asymptomatic but may still spread the infection to others. Infection spreads primarily through contact with fecal material, most often on the hands.
- *Preventive measures*: Patients must take antibiotics only as prescribed and should avoid asking for unnecessary antibiotic prescriptions. Careful hand washing by the patient and caregivers is essential.

Transmission of Hepatitis C and Transmission Prevention

Hepatitis C virus (HCV) binds to receptors on hepatic cells and enters to begin replicating. HCV readily mutates, which helps it to evade the host's immune response. There is no vaccine. HCV is transmitted directly through blood or items, such as shared needles, contaminated with blood. It can also be spread by sexual contact, tattooing, and piercing. HCV causes an acute infection (first 6 months), but 75-85% develop chronic infection. Patients are also at increased risk of liver cancer, and HCV is the primary reasons for liver transplants. Nosocomial infections are similar to HBV and related to contaminated blood sampling equipment, multidose vials, improperly sterilized equipment, and breakdown in infection control methods, so proper use of contact precautions is essential as is educating patients about avoidance of sharing needles and importance of using condoms. New antiviral treatments are up to 90% effective in treating HCV, but there are 6 HCV genotypes, and different medications target different genotypes. Options include Daklinza®, Zepatier®, Mavyret®, Harvoni®, and Technivie®.

CGRN Practice Test

1. Which of the following dairy products is MOST LIKELY to contain the least lactose for those who are lactose intolerant?

   1. Whole milk
   2. Cheese
   3. Regular whole-fat yogurt
   4. Greek-style whole-fat yogurt

2. Unless otherwise specified by manufacturer, multi-use vials that have been accessed and used should be discarded within which of the following time periods?

   1. One week
   2. 14 days
   3. 28 days
   4. 60 days

3. Which of the following is a reversal agent for excessive sedation of a patient who has received a benzodiazepine?

   1. Atropine
   2. Romazicon (Flumazenil®)
   3. Naloxone (Narcan®)
   4. N-acetylcysteine

4. Following an esophagoscopy to obtain a biopsy of the thoracic esophagus, which of the following symptoms MOST indicates the need for emergent care for perforation?

   1. Chest pain, dysphagia, and tachycardia
   2. Mild cough and sore throat
   3. Nausea and vomiting
   4. Local discomfort but no systemic response

5. A 76-year-old female ate *E. coli* (O157:H7) contaminated vegetables and developed abdominal cramps and non-bloody diarrhea for 48 hours after which the diarrhea became bloody for 4 days. The patient is MOST at risk for developing which of the following?

   1. Intestinal necrosis
   2. Small bowel obstruction
   3. Intestinal perforation
   4. Hemolytic uremic syndrome

6. A patient taking metoclopramide has been prescribed haloperidol. For which of the following does this drug combination put the patient at increased risk?

   1. Tachycardia
   2. Tardive dyskinesia
   3. Excessive sedation
   4. GI bleeding

7. If a patient scheduled for a colonoscopy has a nose stud and enclosed lip ring, which of the following actions is appropriate?

    1. Remove the lip ring and tape the nose stud securely
    2. Leave both in place
    3. Remove both prior to the procedure
    4. Remove the nose stud but leave the lip ring in place

8. Cancer of the colon and rectum is primarily which of the following types of cancer?

    1. Adenocarcinoma
    2. Sarcoma
    3. Lymphoma
    4. Melanoma

9. According to the WHO three-step ladder approach to pain management, if a patient's abdominal pain associated with colon cancer varies from 4 to 8 on the pain scale, at which of the following steps should pain control be initiated?

    1. Step 1
    2. Step 2
    3. Step 3
    4. Whichever step is appropriate at the time of initiation

10. How soon after collection should duodenal aspirate be transported to the laboratory?

    1. Immediately
    2. Within 2 hours
    3. Within 4 hours
    4. Within 24 hours

11. The gastroenterology unit has experienced an outbreak of *Clostridium difficile* infections involving 10 patients over a 2-week period. In order to reduce further transmission of the infection, on which of the following should the staff should concentrate efforts?

    1. Antibiotic stewardship
    2. Contact precautions/hand hygiene
    3. Testing patient stool specimens
    4. Limiting patient contacts

12. A patient with Crohn's disease is to begin treatment with infliximab, a biologic response modifier. For which of the following should the patient be tested prior to beginning treatment?

    1. Anemia
    2. Diabetes and hepatitis C
    3. TB and hepatitis B
    4. Hepatitis A and B

13. A Navajo patient tells the nurse that he has "ghost sickness." Which of the following is the MOST appropriate response?

    1. "There is no such disease."
    2. "What do you mean?"
    3. "Is that a common name for a real illness?"
    4. "How does ghost sickness make you feel?"

14. Doppler ultrasound is used primarily to assess which of the following?

    1. Size and shape
    2. Blood flow
    3. Function
    4. Consistency (air-filled, fluid-filled)

15. The nurse is using the BVMGR (beliefs, values, meanings, goals, and relationships) rubric for implementing spiritual care. To which of the following do these aspects apply?

    1. The nurse
    2. The culture
    3. The patient
    4. The organization

16. Capsule endoscopy is used primarily to examine which part of the gastrointestinal tract?

    1. Small intestine
    2. Large intestine
    3. Stomach
    4. Esophagus

17. Which of the following increases the risk of aspiration for a patient receiving NG feedings?

    1. Head elevated at 45 degree
    2. Continuous feeding
    3. Young age
    4. History of diabetes mellitus

18. A patient complains of increasing abdominal pain and has been passing 3 to 4 sticky, black foul-smelling stools for 4 days and exhibits postural hypotension, hemoglobin of 9.2 mg/dL, and hematocrit of 28%. Which of the following should the nurse suspect?

    1. Iron deficiency anemia and intestinal perforation
    2. Hemolytic anemia and gastritis
    3. Iron deficiency anemia and upper GI bleeding
    4. Iron deficiency anemia and lower GI bleeding

19. A patient has been prescribed antibiotic therapy and probiotics to help to maintain intestinal flora. Which of the following statements BEST describes the appropriate administration?

    1. The antibiotic and the probiotics should be taken simultaneously
    2. The antibiotic and the probiotics should be taken at least 2 hours apart
    3. The probiotics should be started only after completing the antibiotic
    4. The probiotics should be taken for 2 days before beginning the antibiotic

20. The nurse hears a patient's physician complaining that a patient is "difficult and impatient," and the nurse tells the physician that the patient is very frightened and acting defensively. Which of the followings aspects of care is the nurse exhibiting?

    1. Advocacy
    2. Patient equality
    3. Human dignity preservation
    4. Caring practice

21. Imaging shows that a patient has an intestinal obstruction from a cancerous lesion at the duodenum. The patient is MOST likely to exhibit which of the following signs and symptoms?

    1. Copious emesis of undigested food, succession splashing bowel sounds, but absence of abdominal pain or distention

    2. Moderate emesis, hyperactive bowel sounds, and upper abdominal pain

    3. Moderate abdominal distention, colicky cramping, and hyperactive bowel sounds

    4. Marked abdominal distention, some emesis (late), borborygmi, and colicky pain in central and lower abdomen

22. Which of the following herbal preparations should the nurse advise a patient to avoid when taking immunosuppressant drugs?

    1. Melatonin

    2. St. John's wort

    3. Chamomile

    4. Curcumin

23. If two grounding pads (AKA return electrodes) are utilized during a procedure involving electrical cautery, which of the following is a correct placement?

    1. Upper thigh and lower thigh

    2. Left thigh and right calf

    3. Right upper thigh and left upper thigh

    4. Anterior thigh and posterior thigh

24. When reviewing medications for a patient with cirrhosis, the nurse must consider that the liver disease may MOST affect which of the following?

    1. Absorption

    2. Metabolism

    3. Distribution

    4. Excretion

25. Ensuring that a patient has given informed consent and understands his or her rights and all of the risks and benefits of a procedure or treatment supports which of the following ethical principles?

    1. Beneficence

    2. Nonmaleficence

    3. Justice

    4. Autonomy

26. A patient with inflammatory bowel disease has periodic bouts of severe diarrhea but is unsure of the cause. Which of the following should the nurse advise the patient to do to try to resolve the problem?

    1. Maintain a food diary

    2. Avoid all milk products

    3. Increase fat in diet

    4. Increase fiber in diet

27. Absorption of nutrients from the small bowel is often impaired in older adults because of which of the following?

    1. Age-related cellular mutations
    2. Decreased muscular contractility
    3. Narrowing and lengthening of villi
    4. Broadening and shortening of villi

28. A 72-year-old patient has 3 polyps removed during a routine colonoscopy. Which of the following types of polyps are precancerous?

    1. Epithelial hyperplastic
    2. Adenomatous
    3. Inflammatory
    4. Submucosal (fibroma)

29. The nurse is educating a patient who is to be discharged after surgery to remove a cancerous lesion of the colon and create a colostomy. Which of the following foods may cause a noticeable odor?

    1. Green beans, raw fruits, spicy foods, and spinach
    2. Popcorn, seeds, raw vegetables, and corn
    3. Fish, eggs, onions, broccoli, and cabbage
    4. Beans, carbonated beverages, strong cheeses, and sprouts

30. Following a colonoscopy with removal of polyps, a patient developed abdominal pain with elevated temperature, WBC count and C-reactive protein. Which of the following interventions does the nurse anticipate initially?

    1. Abdominal CT
    2. Repeat colonoscopy
    3. Antibiotic therapy
    4. Exploratory laparotomy

31. If a patient develops an infection with a multi-drug resistant organism (MDRO), the nurse anticipates that the patient's history will show which of the following?

    1. Auto-immune disorder
    2. Pneumonia
    3. Diabetes mellitus
    4. Prior antibiotic use

32. The standard triple therapy for *H. pylori*-associated peptic ulcer disease includes a proton pump inhibitor BID, clarithromycin 500 mg BID, and which of the following?

    1. Bismuth subcitrate potassium 140 mg qd
    2. H-2 receptor antagonist
    3. Amoxicillin 1 g BID
    4. Misoprostol 200 mcg QID

33. When lifting an item, which of the muscles should be used?

    1. The muscles in the legs
    2. The muscles in the arm
    3. The muscles in the lower back
    4. The muscles in the upper back and shoulders

34. When palpating a patient's abdomen, a positive Murphy's sign (sudden holding of breath with RUQ palpation) MOST LIKELY indicates which of the following?
1. Appendicitis
2. Cholecystitis
3. Choledocholithiasis
4. Duodenal ulcer

35. If a patient is receiving methotrexate for maintenance treatment of Crohn's disease, which laboratory tests should be routinely monitored?
1. CBC and renal function tests
2. CBC and sed rate
3. CBC and renal and liver function tests
4. CBC and pancreatic enzymes

36. A patient presents with symptoms consistent with diverticulosis. Which of the following imaging techniques does the nurse anticipate will be used to confirm the diagnosis?
1. Colonic contrast studies
2. Colonoscopy
3. Abdominal CT
4. Abdominal ultrasound

37. A patient comes to the emergency department with slight jaundice and complaining of clay-colored stools and flu-like symptom. Which of the following are the primary tests that screen for suspected hepatitis?
1. ALT and AST
2. CBC and differential
3. Bilirubin and LDH
3. Total protein and serum ammonia

38. Environmental surfaces have been implicated in transmission of which of the following healthcare-associated pathogens?
1. Clostridium difficile only
2. Clostridium difficile and norovirus only
3. Methicillin-resistant Staphylococcus aureus only
4. Clostridium difficile, norovirus, and Staphylococcus aureus/MRSA

39. Under the Spaulding system, which of the following is classified as a semi-critical item when considering methods for sterilization/disinfection?
1. Surgical instrument
2. Prosthetic implant
3. Endoscope
4. Blood pressure cuff

40. Following removal of the esophagogastroduodenoscopy tube, the patient begins to cough violently and appears cyanotic. Which of the following is the MOST appropriate initial intervention?

1. Turn patient onto one side
2. Suction airway and increase supplemental oxygen
3. Reverse sedation
4. Encourage deep breathing and coughing

41. Which of the following is the CDC-recommended method of routine hand hygiene?

1. Wearing gloves
2. Washing with soap and water
3. Using alcohol-based hand rubs
4. Using chlorhexidine scrubs

42. In regards to reprocessing of single-use devices, the CMS recommends which of the following?

1. No reprocessing
2. In-house reprocessing
3. Reprocessing of class I devices only
4. Use of third-party reprocessors

43. Which of the following is the incubation period for foodborne illness caused by *Salmonella* spp.?

1. 1 to 6 hours
2. 1 to 3 days
3. 12 to 48 hours
4. 28 days

44. Constipation is usually defined as which of the following?

1. Fewer than 7 stools per week
2. Fewer than 5 stools per week
3. Fewer than 3 stools per week
4. Fewer than 2 stools per week

45. Which of the following is MOST indicated for an inactive patient who has been taking laxatives long-term to treat chronic bouts of constipation and fecal impaction?

1. Stool softeners
2. High fiber diet
3. Exercise program
4. Bowel retraining

46. A patient is receiving enteral feedings. Which of the following is MOST LIKELY to contribute to diarrhea?

1. Cold formula
2. Warm formula
3. Hypo-osmolar formula
4. Continuous feeding

47. When undergoing a bowel transit time test, how soon after ingesting markers should the patient return for radiographs?

    1. 24 hours
    2. 2 days
    3. 4 days
    4. 5 days

48. A patient has developed acne, weight gain, mood swings, and hyperglycemia. Which of the following drugs is MOST LIKELY to cause these symptoms?

    1. Balsalazide (Aminosalicylate)
    2. Azathioprine (Immunomodulator)
    3. Prednisone (Corticosteroid)
    4. Infliximab (Biologic)

49. Which of the following BEST describes the action of omeprazole (Prilosec®)?

    1. Suppresses secretion of gastric acids
    2. Speeds gastric emptying
    3. Slows intestinal motility
    4. Neutralizes gastric secretions

50. Which of the following is the MOST common cause of fecal incontinence?

    1. Chronic diarrhea
    2. Fecal impaction
    3. Neurological impairment
    4. Laxative abuse

51. In a bowel diary, the Bristol Stool Form Scale is used for which of the following?

    1. To describe the frequency of incontinence
    2. To differentiate between defecation and incontinence
    3. To describe the amount of stool
    4. To describe the type of stool

52. A patient has been dieting but complains that she has developed chronic diarrhea. Which of the following items recorded in the patient's food diary is MOST LIKELY to cause diarrhea?

    1. Dietetic hard candy
    2. Broccoli
    3. Cottage cheese
    4. Hard-boiled eggs

53. A patient has prescriptions from four different doctors and admits to taking additional "pills" but can't recall which ones and gives conflicting information regarding the dosage and frequency of the different medications. Which of the following do these findings MOST LIKELY indicate?

    1. Dementia
    2. Overdose
    3. Polypharmacy
    4. Drug-seeking behavior

54. Which of the following is the MOST common cause of upper GI bleeding?

    1. Neoplasm
    2. Peptic ulcer disease
    3. Post-procedural trauma
    4. Esophageal varices

55. The nurse is teaching a patient to care for a PEG feeding tube. Which of the following should the nurse advise the patient to do to avoid dumping syndrome?

    1. Administer refrigerated formula
    2. Increase rate of instillation
    3. Stay in semi-Fowler's position for one hour after feedings
    4. Increase volume of water used to flush tube before and after feedings

56. The Health Insurance Portability and Accountability Act (HIPAA) regulates which of the following?

    1. Rights of the individual related to privacy of health information
    2. Transfer of patients from one facility to another
    3. Medical trials
    4. Workplace safety

57. A 69-year-old patient is learning to care for a colostomy but is quite tense and becomes confused about the sequence of actions required. Which of the following is the MOST appropriate teaching strategy?

    1. Teach a family member or caregiver to do colostomy care
    2. Break the tasks into small steps and teach sequentially
    3. Review the entire procedure 3 or 4 times before patient participates
    4. Suggest patient try to relax and concentrate

58. A patient complains of a history of nausea and burning and stabbing epigastric pain, relieved for short periods by antacids or intake of food, and a urea breath test is positive. These findings MOST LIKELY indicate which of the following?

    1. Esophagitis
    2. Gastritis and *Salmonella* infection
    3. Reflux
    4. Duodenal ulcer and *Helicobacter pylori* infection

59. A 60-year old male has had yearly negative fecal occult blood tests for 10 years. How frequently should the patient have a colonoscopy?

    1. Every year
    2. Every 5 years
    3. Every 10 years
    4. Every 2 years until age 70

60. Which of the following is a long double-lumen tube inserted into the small intestine for drainage and decompression?

    1. Salem sump
    2. Miller-Abbott
    3. Cantor
    4. Levin

61. A patient has had severe watery diarrhea and vomiting for 48 hours. Which electrolyte imbalance is MOST LIKELY to occur?

    1. Hypernatremia
    2. Hyponatremia
    3. Hypercalcemia
    4. Hypocalcemia

62. Most absorption of nutrients occurs in which of the following?

    1. Stomach
    2. Duodenum
    3. Jejunum and ileum
    4. Large intestine

63. Which of the following types of laxatives/cathartics is MOST recommended for chronic constipation?

    1. Stimulant
    2. Lubricant
    3. Emollient/wetting
    4. Bulk-forming

64. How long after PEG is performed is the tract usually mature and well-healed enough for placement of a balloon gastrostomy (G-tube)?

    1. 4 to 7 days
    2. 2 to 4 weeks
    3. 1 to 2 months
    4. 3 to 4 months

65. Which of the following is the correct response if, in the initial period after surgery for a colostomy, the stoma appears dull and blue-tinged?

    1. Notify the physician
    2. Observe for further changes
    3. No response needed, as this is normal finding
    4. Provide patient with nasal oxygen

66. When irrigating a Kock pouch to improve drainage postoperatively, what is the maximal amount of fluid that should be instilled at one time?

    1. ≤1000 mL
    2. ≤500 mL
    3. ≤100 mL
    4. ≤40 mL

67. How soon after collection must an unpreserved stool be tested for ova and parasites?

    1. 30 minutes
    2. 60 minutes
    3. 2 hours
    4. 4 hours

68. What of the following is the MOST LIKELY cause when a patient with an ileo-anal pouch develops a sudden increase in the frequency of stools as well as bloody diarrhea, fever, and fecal incontinence?

    1. Peritonitis
    2. Pouchitis
    3. Anastomotic leak
    4. Fistula formation

69. When checking aspirant from a J-PEG tube, which pH value is consistent with possible gastric migration?

    1. 0 to 4
    2. >6
    3. <6
    4. >7.5

70. Which of the following is the first goal in management of enterocutaneous fistula?

    1. Control fluid and electrolyte imbalance
    2. Initiate parenteral nutrition
    3. Decrease discharge
    4. Complete surgical repair

71. Which of the following complications outside of the gastrointestinal tract is MOST common with patients with inflammatory bowel disease?

    1. Osteoporosis
    2. Fibromyalgia
    3. Migraines
    4. Anemia

72. How far away from the skin surface should the external fixation device of a PEG tube be placed to prevent buried bumper syndrome?

    1. 1 to 2 cm
    2. 2 to 3 cm
    3. 4 to 5 cm
    4. Flush with the skin

73. When inserting a balloon replacement gastrostomy tube, in which of the following positions should the nurse place the patient?

    1. Flat supine
    2. Head of bed elevated 30 degrees
    3. Head of bed elevated 45 degrees
    4. Head of bed elevated 60 degrees

74. Which of the following is a legal document that specifically designates someone to make decisions regarding medical and end-of-life care if a patient is mentally incompetent?

    1. Advance directive
    2. Do-not-resuscitate order
    3. Durable Power of Attorney
    4. General Power of Attorney

75. A 30-year-old patient with Crohn's disease is disabled and uninsured because of illness but unable to afford medications to control the disease. Which of the following is the MOST LIKELY source of financial assistance?

    1. Medicaid
    2. Drug companies
    3. Community agency
    4. Salvation Army

76. With cardiac arrest, immediate defibrillation is indicated for which of the following?

    1. Pulseless electrical activity (PEA)
    2. Asystole
    3. Ventricular fibrillation/tachycardia (VF/VT)
    4. All cardiac abnormalities

77. A patient is scheduled the next day for an abdominal ultrasound to evaluate the liver, pancreas, and bile ducts. Which of the following preparations does the nurse anticipate?

    1. No special preparations
    2. Fat-free dinner and NPO after midnight
    3. Drink 6 glasses of water 60 minutes before the ultrasound
    4. NPO after midnight

78. A 70-year-old patient has advanced gastric carcinoma. Which of the following criteria makes the patient eligible for Hospice care?

    1. The patient has stopped curative treatments but life expectancy is unclear
    2. The patient continues curative treatment and life expectancy is 4 months
    3. The patient has only palliative care and life expectancy is 12 months
    4. The patient has stopped curative treatments and life expectancy is 6 months

79. Which of the following is the MOST common site for obstructions of the small intestine?

    1. Duodenum
    2. Jejunum
    3. Ileum
    4. Ileocecal junction

80. Following cholecystectomy, a patient develops paralytic ileus. Which of the following interventions does the nurse anticipate?

    1. Insertion of NG tube and decompression
    2. Surgical intervention
    3. Antibiotics and antispasmodics
    4. Antibiotics and enteral feedings

81. Which of the following acid-base disorders is MOST common with acute mesenteric ischemia?

    1. Respiratory alkalosis
    2. Respiratory acidosis
    3. Metabolic alkalosis
    4. Metabolic acidosis

82. If bacteria, such as *Escherichia coli,* produce extended spectrum beta lactamase (ESBL), which of the following should the nurse anticipate?

    1. The bacteria will respond rapidly to antibiotics
    2. The bacteria will be resistant to multiple antibiotics
    3. The bacteria will become neutralized
    4. The bacteria will mutate into a more virulent form

83. Which of the following forms of anesthesia is MOST commonly used when a patient requires removal of a foreign object from the rectum?

    1. Benzodiazepine and opioid
    2. Perianal block
    3. Topical lidocaine
    4. General anesthesia

84. Which of the following is the MOST common positioning for a patient who is to undergo a rigid sigmoidoscopy for sigmoid volvulus?

    1. Lithotomy
    2. Prone, knee-chest
    3. Left lateral (Sims)
    4. Right lateral

85. If a patient has received midazolam for an endoscopic procedure, how soon after administration does the peak effect occur?

    1. 60 seconds.
    2. 3 to 5 minutes.
    3. 5 to 8 minutes.
    4. 10 minutes.

86. A patient is to receive antibiotic prophylaxis for placement of PEG tube. When should the antibiotic be administered?

    1. 30 minutes before the procedure
    2. during the procedure
    3. immediately after the procedure
    4. within 60 minutes after the procedure

87. According to Health.gov recommendations for fiber intake, how many grams of fiber should be consumed for each 1000 calories?

    1. 10
    2. 14
    3. 20
    4. 24

88. Within 90 seconds of receiving midazolam for an endoscopic procedure, the patient exhibits signs of anaphylaxis with bronchospasm and severe hypotension. Which of the following is the correct INITIAL emergent response?

    1. Administer epinephrine
    2. Administer antihistamine
    3. Administer corticosteroid
    4. Administer romazicon (Flumazenil®)

89. A stool specimen to test for *Clostridium difficile* may be held under refrigeration prior to testing for how long?

    1. 4 hours
    2. 24 hours
    3. 3 days
    4. 5 days

90. The esophageal pH probe is usually left in place for what duration of time?

    1. 4 hours
    2. 12 hours
    3. 24 hours
    4. 36 hours

91. Once a rubber band ligation is carried out for a second-degree hemorrhoid, within how many days does the tissue usually slough off.

    1. One day
    2. 1 to 3 days
    3. 3 to 5 days
    4. 7 to 14 days

92. If using the FAITH mnemonic as a guide to a spiritual assessment, the H stands for which of the following?

    1. Help
    2. Hope
    3. History
    4. Health

93. Which of the following is the MOST common reason for sexual dysfunction after an ileostomy/colostomy?

    1. Nerve damage
    2. Medications
    3. Psychological inhibitions
    4. Hormonal changes

94. Patients who have had bariatric surgery should generally limit total meal size to which of the following?

    1. Less than one-half cup
    2. Less than one cup
    3. Less than one and a half cups
    4. Less than two cups

95. If administering a bolus feeding of 400 mL per a gastrostomy tube, the feeding should generally be given over which of the following durations?

    1. 1 to 2 minutes
    2. 3 to 8 minutes
    3. 10 to 15 minutes
    4. 20 to 30 minutes

96. Following gastric surgery with removal of the pylorus, a patient develops bile reflux gastritis/esophagitis. Which of the following treatments is MOST indicated?

1. Cholestyramine (Questran®)
2. Ranitidine (Zantac®)
3. Metoclopramide (Reglan®)
4. Cimetadine (Tagamet®)

97. Which of the following is a cause of exudative diarrhea?

1. Bacterial toxins
2. Intestinal hemorrhage or pancreatic impairment
3. Decreased serum albumin
4. Radiation or chemotherapy

98. In order to prevent contracting an *Escherichia coli* infection from eating contaminated meat, all ground beef should be cooked to at least which of the following temperatures?

1. 145° F
2. 160° F
3. 175° F
4. 190° F

99. A hospitalized patient with persistent watery diarrhea is to use the Flexi-seal Fecal Management System®. Which of the following is the correct procedure after the cuff is inserted into the rectum?

1. Gently tug on the device to automatically inflate the cuff
2. Use a syringe to withdraw air from the cuff
3. Use a syringe to fill with 45 mL air
4. Use a syringe to fill with 45 mL water

100. Which of the following complications is MOST LIKELY to occur with ulcerative colitis?

1. Abscess
2. Fistula
3. Fissure
4. Obstruction

101. Patients with celiac disease must be advised to avoid foods that contain which of the following?

1. Lactose
2. Purines
3. Gluten
4. Food additives

102. Which of the following ethnic groups have the highest prevalence of ulcerative colitis?

1. African Americans
2. Middle Easterners
3. Asians and Hispanics
4. Caucasians and Ashkenazi Jews

103. A 40-year-old patient with a history of Chagas disease reports increasing dysphagia, cough, regurgitation, drooling, and heartburn. Which of the following is the MOST LIKELY cause?

    1. GERD
    2. Gastric ulcer
    3. Megaesophagus
    4. Esophagitis

104. Which of the following is the drug of choice to treat *Giardia* infection?

    1. Metronidazole
    2. Iodoquinol
    3. Tetracycline
    4. Diloxanide furoate

105. Which of the following is the MOST common test for pinworms?

    1. Stool specimen
    2. Cellophane test
    3. Antibody test
    4. C-reactive protein

106. For moderate sedation, ASA guidelines require monitoring of which of the following?

    1. ECG and pulse oximetry
    2. EEG
    3. ECG
    4. Capnography and pulse oximetry

107. Which of the following is the primary reason for liver transplants?

    1. Hepatitis A
    2. Hepatitis B
    3. Hepatitis C
    4. Hepatitis D

108. Which of the following is the MOST common carbapenem-resistant Enterobacteriaceae (CRE) in the United States?

    1. *Klebsiella pneumoniae* carbapenemase (KPC)
    2. New Delhi Metallo-beta-lactamase (NDM-1)
    3. Verona Integron-Mediated Metallo-beta-lactamase (VIM)
    4. *Escherichia coli* carbapenemase (ECC)

109. When examining the abdomen for bowel sounds, for how long should the nurse auscultate before determining bowel sounds are absent?

    1. 1 minute
    2. 2 minutes
    3. 3 minutes
    4. 5 minutes

110. A patient who has recently had formation of an ileostomy suffers from disturbed body image. Which of the following is the BEST nursing intervention?

1. Avoid discussing the colostomy
2. Encourage the patient to verbalize feelings
3. Focus on the positives
4. Provide information about colostomy care

111. A male patient complains of decreased libido and increasing erectile dysfunction. Which of the following OTC drugs/supplements may be contributing?

1. Cimetidine (Tagamet®)
2. Vitamin D
3. Acetaminophen
4. Docusate

112. Which of the following disinfectants can provide high-level disinfection?

1. Isopropyl alcohol 70%
2. Sodium hypochlorite 6.15%
3. Glutaraldehyde 2%
4. Iodophor germicidal detergent

113. Which of the following is the primary treatment for a norovirus infection?

1. Antibiotics
2. Antivirals
3. Antiemetics and antidiarrheals
4. Supportive care and fluids

114. In which of the following parts of the bowel are fats, proteins, and carbohydrates absorbed?

1. Jejunum
2. Duodenum
3. Ileum
4. Throughout the small bowel

115. If a patient has persistent dyspepsia/indigestion, which type of food is likely to cause the MOST discomfort?

1. Proteins
2. Carbohydrates
3. Fats
4. All cause similar reactions

116. If assisting with an endoscopic procedure, which of the following PPE should the nurse expect to wear?

1. Gown and gloves
2. Gown, gloves, and face mask
3. Gown, gloves and eye guard
4. Full surgical attire

117. Which of the following is a common age-related change in the stomach?

1. Increased secretion of gastric acids
2. Decreased production of hydrochloric acid
3. Increased gastric motility and emptying
4. Increased secretion of digestive enzymes

118. What distance from the anus can a flexible sigmoidoscope examine?

1. 25 cm/10 inches
2. 45-50 cm/16-20 inches
3. 50-75 cm/20-30 inches
4. 75-100 cm/30-40 9nches

119. During a gastroscopy, the patient becomes very faint and light-headed and experiences hypotension, bradycardia, and diaphoresis. Which of the following is MOST LIKELY the cause of these symptoms?

1. Vasovagal response
2. Aspiration
3. Oversedation
4. Perforation

120. If a patient has a hiatal hernia, what information is important to prevent symptoms?

1. Avoid reclining for 30 minutes after meals
2. Use two pillows when sleeping
3. Eat small frequent meals
4. Take frequent antacids

121. If a chemical spill occurs, which of the following is the BEST initial resource to determine what actions to take?

1. Manufacturer's hotline
2. Poison center
3. Supervisor
4. Material Data Safety Sheet (MDSS)

122. Which of the following is the primary purpose of a "time-out" prior to beginning a procedure?

1. To ensure all members of the team are present
2. To prevent surgical/procedural errors
3. To help the team members relax
4. To remind team members of their responsibilities

123. Which of the following is the correct method of administration of vedolizumab (ENTYVIO®), a biologic drug used to treat IBS?

1. Bolus over 1 minute
2. Bolus over 5 minutes
3. Infusion over 15 minutes
4. Infusion over 30 minutes

124. The nurse is to mix two medications in one syringe for administration and injects air into vial A and then vial B. Which of the following is the next step?

    1. Obtain a new needle and syringe
    2. Withdraw medication from vial A
    3. Withdraw medication from vial B
    4. Withdraw medication from either vial A or vial B

125. Gastric aspirate must be neutralized with bicarbonate within which of the following durations after collection?

    1. 30 minutes
    2. 60 minutes
    3. 4 hours
    4. 8 hours

126. A 28-year-old woman who had gastric bypass surgery (Roux-en-Y) experiences bloating, abdominal cramping, nausea, and vomiting within minutes after eating. Her typical meal consists of a small potato, 3 ounces of meat, half a slice of white bread, half a banana, a small piece of cake, and 8 ounces of sweetened iced tea. Which of the following is indicated as an initial treatment?

    1. Acarbose to delay carbohydrate absorption
    2. Octreotide to slow intestinal emptying
    3. Increased protein, reduced carbohydrates, and avoiding drinking during meals
    4. Decreased protein, increased carbohydrates, and a glass of juice or milk during meals

127. Prior to a nasogastric tube feeding, a pH check of aspirant reveals a pH of 8. This most likely indicates that the tube tip is in the

    1. stomach.
    2. respiratory system.
    3. small intestine.
    4. esophagus.

128. As part of a bowel-training program, a patient has a daily scheduled defecation. What is the best time to schedule a bowel movement?

    1. First thing in the morning after arising
    2. At bedtime
    3. 2 hours after a meal
    4. 20 to 30 minutes after a meal

129. Post-infectious irritable bowel syndrome (PI-IBS) is most commonly characterized by which of the following?

    1. Fever
    2. Altered bowel habits with chronic diarrhea
    3. Constipation
    4. Flu-like symptoms

130. In conducting research, which of the following types of studies represents one in which those with a condition (such as infection) are compared to those without the condition?

    1. Retrospective cohort study
    2. Prospective cohort study
    3. Case control study
    4. Cross-sectional study

131. Which of the following is a typical symptom associated with rectoceles?

    1. Chronic constipation
    2. Chronic diarrhea
    3. Pulling sensation in pelvic area
    4. Vaginal discharge

132. A patient being treated for a gastric ulcer has been stable on medications. Which of the following indicates a possible emergent situation that the nurse should report to the physician immediately?

    1. Inability to sleep well and generalized anxiety
    2. Periodic epigastric pain (heartburn) relieved by medications
    3. Nausea after taking prescribed antibiotics
    4. Increasing back and epigastric pain unrelieved by medications

133. Peristomal abscess is most commonly associated with which of the following conditions?

    1. Crohn's disease
    2. Systemic bacterial infection
    3. Paralytic ileus
    4. Ulcerative colitis

134. Which of the following histamine receptor antagonists should those taking oral contraceptive agents or estrogen avoid?

    1. Ranitidine (brand name Zantac)
    2. Famotidine (brand name Pepcid)
    3. Cimetidine (brand name Tagamet)
    4. Nizatidine (brand name Axid)

135. Which test measures the pressure of the anal sphincter muscles, degree of rectal sensation, and neural reflexes?

    1. Anal wink
    2. Bulbocavernosus reflex
    3. Endoanal ultrasound
    4. Anal manometry

136. Which provision of the National Patient Safety Goals governs getting laboratory test results to the appropriate staff person on time?

    1. Improving staff communication
    2. Identifying patients correctly
    3. Identifying patient safety risks
    4. Preventing surgical mistakes

137. A patient is scheduled for anal sphincter electromyography. Which of the patient's medications should be stopped prior to the EMG?

    1. Stool softener
    2. Anticholinergic
    3. Antibiotic
    4. Warfarin

138. Which of the following is most important to avoid fluid and electrolyte imbalance with an ileostomy?

    1. Increase intake of high fiber foods to slow absorption
    2. Increase intake of water with diarrhea
    3. Take routine antidiarrheal medication
    4. Monitor intake and output

139. A patient with a loop ileostomy and a retained distal segment of bowel has copious anal discharge of mucous. Which of the following is the most likely cause?

    1. Normal mucous production
    2. Diversion colitis
    3. Anastomotic leak
    4. Fluid and electrolyte imbalance

140. According to the ANA Nursing Code of Ethics, nurses must support a patient's autonomy and self-determination. A 44-year-old Asian woman states a treatment preference but plans to leave the decision to family members. Which of the following actions is correct?

    1. Recognize that cultural values regarding individualism vary and respect the patient's right to be guided by family
    2. Try to convince the patient to assert herself
    3. Tell the family that the patient should be the one to make the decision
    4. Ask the ethics committee to intervene

141. The nurse is teaching a 50-year old woman with a colostomy to do irrigations and has prepared written directions and a video, but the patient ignores them and picks up the equipment and looks at each part, trying to figure it out. The patient's learning style is probably which of the following?

    1. Auditory
    2. Visual
    3. Kinesthetic
    4. Mixed

142. A patient who receives multiple transfusions for GI bleeding with citrated blood products must be monitored closely for which of the following?

    1. Hyponatremia
    2. Hypomagnesemia
    3. Hypokalemia
    4. Hypocalcemia

143. The patient has a percutaneous endoscopic gastrostomy (PEG) and has developed leakage about the tube. What initial intervention is indicated?

    1. Check balloon to ensure adequate inflation
    2. Stabilize the tube with the bumper and external stabilizer
    3. Replace tube
    4. Apply barrier ointment

144. For which of the following is a positive Murphy's sign an aid in diagnosis?

    1. Differentiating cholecystitis from choledocholithiasis
    2. Diagnosing cholecystitis in geriatric patients
    3. Diagnosing pancreatitis
    4. Differentiating ascending cholangitis from pancreatitis

145. Which of the following is a contraindication for upper GI endoscopy?

    1. Reflux disease
    2. Esophageal diverticulum
    3. Barrett esophagus
    4. Caustic esophageal injury

146. In evidence-based research, what does persistent erratic findings in tracking and trending suggest?

    1. Changes in patient population requiring changes in processes of care
    2. Errors in statistical analysis of processes of care
    3. Normal day-to-day variations in processes of care
    4. Inconsistent or inadequate processes of care

147. Prior to beginning an invasive procedure, which of the following is most important for infection control?

    1. Completing a safety pre-procedure checklist
    2. Ensuring correct patient, correct procedure
    3. Checking patient records to make sure pre-procedure orders have been carried out
    4. Providing adequate patient education

148. A 25-year-old woman who required an ileostomy refuses to look at the stoma or participate in care postoperatively. Which of the following is the most likely to promote cooperation?

    1. Refer patient to a psychologist
    2. Ask family to intervene
    3. Arrange visit with a recovered ostomate
    4. Advise patient of the importance of self-care

149. Over-transfusing must be avoided with treatment for esophageal variceal hemorrhage for which of the following reasons?

    1. Underlying coagulopathy
    2. Increased central and portal venous pressures
    3. Generalized edema
    4. Third-space shift

150. Which of the following laboratory findings 36 hours after hospital admission is predictive of severe pancreatitis?

    1. Serum calcium greater than 8 mg/dL (2.0 mmol/L)
    2. BUN decrease less than 5 mg/dL
    3. Decrease in hematocrit greater than 10%
    4. PO_2 less than 80 mm Hg

151. Which of the following actions is an example of Standard I, Quality of Practice, in Standards of Professional Performance of the Standards of Clinical Practice and Role Delineation for Certified Gastroenterology Nurses?

    1. Participating in peer review
    2. Collecting data regarding quality of care
    3. Demonstrating commitment to lifelong learning
    4. Mentoring

152. Which of the following is the first method to use to clear a blockage in an endoscope's air channel?

    1. Flush with water with a small syringe (1 to 5 mL)
    2. Flush with water with a large syringe (50 mL)
    3. Flush with air
    4. Remove tube and cleanse with fine wire

153. Which of the following may interfere with the results of the urea breath test and fecal antigen assay for *H. pylori* infection?

    1. Antacids
    2. Proton pump inhibitors
    3. Anticoagulants
    4. Histamine receptor antagonists.

154. Which type of diet is usually recommended for those with chronic pancreatitis?

    1. Low protein
    2. Low carbohydrate
    3. Low fat
    4. Gluten free

155. For which complications is a patient who has had percutaneous transhepatic cholangiography most at risk?

    1. Bleeding, peritonitis, and septicemia
    2. Bile duct blockage and peritonitis
    3. Intestinal perforation
    4. Allergic reaction to contrast

156. The primary purpose of a transjugular intrahepatic portosystemic shunt (TIPS) is for which of the following?

    1. Preventing hyponatremia
    2. Preventing biliary blockage
    3. Regulating electrolytes
    4. Reducing portal hypertension

157. Which of the following is an appropriate intervention for pain in the right shoulder or scapula after laparoscopic cholecystectomy?

    1. Ice pack to the area for 15 to 20 minutes hourly
    2. Heating pad to the area for 15 to 20 minutes hourly
    3. Range of motion exercises to the right arm
    4. Opioid analgesia

158. Following cholecystectomy, which of the following dietary instructions is appropriate for a patient who experienced preoperative fat intolerance?

    1. Avoid fat in the diet for at least 6 weeks
    2. Add fat into the diet with no restrictions
    3. Add fat into the diet in small increments
    4. Stay on a low fat diet indefinitely

159. For colorectal screening, how often should a patient have a fecal occult blood test done?

    1. Every 10 years
    2. Every 5 years
    3. When symptoms arise
    4. Every year

160. When marking a nasoenteric tube for an adult patient prior to insertion for enteric feedings, what measurements are needed?

    1. Nose to earlobe, earlobe to xiphoid process
    2. Nose to earlobe, earlobe to xiphoid process, plus 6 inches (15 cm)
    3. Nose to earlobe, earlobe to xiphoid process, plus 8 to 10 inches (20-25 cm)
    4. Nose to earlobe, earlobe to xiphoid process, plus 12 to 14 inches (30 t0 38 cm)

161. Following lap-band bariatric surgery, total meal size should be restricted to which of the following?

    1. One-half cup
    2. Less than one cup
    3. One and a half cups
    4. Two cups

162. Which of the following is the most serious complication of enteritis caused by *Escherichia coli,* such as type O157:H7?

    1. Hemolytic uremic syndrome
    2. Iron deficiency anemia
    3. Severe diarrhea
    4. High fever and seizures

163. A patient with Crohn's disease experiences small amounts of diarrhea, increasing abdominal distention and pain, vomiting, and cramping. Which of the following complications is the most likely cause?

    1. Abscess.
    2. Fistula
    3. Colon cancer
    4. Intestinal obstruction

164. A patient receiving total parenteral nutrition (TPN) for inflammatory bowel disease should be monitored every 6 hours for which of the following?

    1. Hemoglobin and hematocrit
    2. Blood glucose level
    3. Blood, urea, nitrogen (BUN)
    4. Electrolytes

165. Which of the following is the most effective method of monitoring small changes in abdominal ascitic fluid?

    1. Observing patient's abdomen while patient is in supine position
    2. Percussing abdomen
    3. Measuring abdominal girth and weighing daily
    4. Assessing abdominal fluid wave

166. Considering placement of a permanent colostomy, which anatomical position is most likely to result in semi-soft, mushy stool?

    1. Ascending colon
    2. Transverse colon
    3. Descending colon
    4. Sigmoid colon

167. What initial cleaning of an endoscope should be completed in the procedure room?

    1. Testing for leakage
    2. Flushing all channels with enzymatic detergent
    3. Rinsing exterior and all channels with clear water
    4. Wiping exterior and flushing the suction channel with water

168. Diabetics well controlled on insulin should make which of the following modifications in insulin dosage on the morning of a scheduled endoscopic procedure?

    1. Omit dosage
    2. Take half a usual dose
    3. Take usual dose
    4. Delay dosage until after procedure

169. Which type of sedation is usually indicated for flexible sigmoidoscopy?

    1. Minimal
    2. Moderate/conscious sedation
    3. Deep sedation
    4. General anesthesia

170. When inserting a small-bore nasogastric tube, which of the following is the best method to verify placement of the tube in the stomach?

    1. Aspirating gastric contents and checking pH
    2. Injecting air and auscultating the gastric region
    3. Taking a chest x-ray
    4. Taking an abdominal x-ray

171. Flumazenil should be available as a reversal agent for which of the following drugs commonly used for endoscopic sedation?

1. Fentanyl
2. Droperidol
3. Midazolam
4. Propofol

172. Which of the following is the best positioning for a patient who is going to undergo a paracentesis?

1. Lying supine with bed flat
2. Side-lying
3. Fowler's position
4. Sitting upright on side of bed or in a chair

173. When using the air insufflation method for bedside postpyloric placement of an enteral feeding tube, which of the following is the best procedure?

1. Inject 350 mL of air and place patient on the right side
2. Administer metoclopramide, 10 mg 10 minutes prior to insertion of tube, followed by injecting 350 mL of air and placing patient on right side
3. Inject 350 mL of air and place patient on the left side
4. Administer an opioid and metoclopramide, 10 mg 10 minutes prior to insertion of tube, followed by injecting 350 mL of air and placing patient on right side

174. When assisting with upper GI endoscopy, which of the following is the best method to prevent aspiration?

1. Position patient properly
2. Pre-medicate patient with antiemetic
3. Ensure patient has been NPO for at least 12 hours prior to procedure
4. Suction all accumulated saliva or emesis during the procedure

175. A patient with stage 2 gastric cancer refuses all treatment because of religious convictions. Which of the following is the most appropriate action?

1. Provide the patient with facts about the disease, treatments, and prognosis
2. Ask family members to intervene
3. Remind the patient that he will die without treatment
4. Refer to a psychologist

Answer Key and Explanations

1. 4. Because Greek-style yogurt is thicker than regular whole-fat yogurt, more of the whey is removed, and the lactose is part of the whey, so those who are lactose intolerant are more likely to tolerate Greek yogurt than other dairy products. Those who are lactose intolerant lack the enzyme needed to digest lactose, resulting in stomach cramps, gas and distention, and diarrhea after eating or drinking dairy products. Some dairy products are now lactose-free, and Lactaid® can be taken to replace the missing enzymes.

2. 3. Unless otherwise specified by manufacturer, multi-use vials that have been accessed and used should be discarded within 28 days. Multi-use vials contain preservatives but can become contaminated with bacteria and provide no protection against viruses. Multi-use vials should be reserved for only one patient whenever possible and should be maintained in a separate space from the treatment area to prevent inadvertent contamination. A new needle and syringe should be used each time the vial is accessed.

3. 2. Romazicon (Flumazenil®) is a reversal agent for excessive sedation of a patient who has received a benzodiazepine although it does not reverse respiratory depression. Romazicon is administered IV with a beginning dose of 0.2 mg over 30 seconds with repeat doses at one-minute intervals as needed. The second dose is 0.3 mg and the third and subsequent doses are 0.5 mg. Epinephrine is used for emergent treatment of asystole, VF, and PEA; naloxone, for opioids; and N-acetylcysteine, for acetaminophen overdose.

4. 1. Following an esophagoscopy to obtain a biopsy of the thoracic esophagus, chest pain, dysphagia, and tachycardia are indications of the need for emergent care for perforation. Onset of fever is often rapid, and Hamann's sign (crunching, rasping precordial sound coinciding with the heartbeat) is positive because of leakage of air to the mediastinum. Perforation is usually confirmed radiologically although CT or endoscopy may be necessary if the perforation cannot be seen on x-ray.

5. 4. If a 76-year-old female ate *E.coli* (O157.H7) contaminated vegetables and developed abdominal cramps and non-bloody diarrhea that persisted for 48 hours after which the diarrhea became bloody for 4 days, the patient is at risk for developing hemolytic uremic syndrome (HUS), which can lead to renal failure. Children under 5 and older adults are most likely to develop HUS. HUS is characterized by microangiopathic hemolytic anemia, thrombocytopenia, and acute renal failure.

6. 2. If a patient taking haloperidol has been prescribed metoclopramide, this drug combination puts the patient at increased risk of developing tardive dyskinesia. Both drugs can cause uncontrollable movement disorders and this combination potentiates the effect and can lead to life-threatening neuroleptic malignant syndrome. The risk of developing tardive dyskinesia with metoclopramide increases with treatment extending beyond 12 weeks. Metoclopramide may also interact with numerous other drugs, including other antipsychotic drugs and phenothiazines.

7. 3. If a patient scheduled for a colonoscopy has a nose stud and enclosed lip ring, they should both be removed prior to the procedure because they pose the risk of trauma and aspiration if they should become dislodged. Nose studs are removed by applying gentle pressure and pulling straight out. Enclosed lip rings are removed by applying pressure inside of the ring to force the ends apart. Barbell-type jewelry has a bead on the end that is unscrewed in a counter-clockwise direction.

8. 1. Cancer of the colon and rectum is primarily (about 95%) adenocarcinoma, which arises in the epithelial lining of the bowel. Adenocarcinomas often develop from a precancerous polyp. Early detection through screening is essential because colorectal cancers may remain essentially asymptomatic until they are advanced and changes in bowel habits or rectal bleeding occurs. Hemorrhage may occur if the tumor invades blood vessels, and obstruction may occur as the mass enlarges.

9. 4. According to the WHO three-step ladder approach to pain management, if a patient's abdominal pain associated with the colon varies from 4 to 8 on the pain scale, pain control should be initiated at whichever step is most appropriate for the level of pain at the time and then may later be adjusted to a higher or lower step. While this is a three-step process, it is not necessary to start all pain control at step one.

10. 1. Duodenal aspirate should be immediately transported to the laboratory because it must be examined within 60 minutes of collection. The aspirate should be collected (at least 2 mL) in a sterile centrifuge tube. Duodenal aspirates may be useful in diagnosing *Giardia duodenalis* and *Strongyloides stercoralis.* Culture and sensitivity may also be done. The specimen should be maintained at room temperature.

11. 2. If the gastroenterology unit has experienced an outbreak of *Clostridium difficile* infections involving 10 patients over a two-week period, in order the reduce transmission of the infection, the nurse and staff members and should concentrate efforts on the utilization of proper contact precautions and hand hygiene as the infection is easily spread through contaminated hands. The spores can remain viable on environmental surfaces for long periods of time. Housekeeping procedures should also be reviewed.

12. 3. If a patient with Crohn's disease is to begin treatment with infliximab or any other biologic response modifier, the patient should be tested for TB and hepatis B prior to beginning treatment. Because the drugs have immunosuppressive qualities, they can result in reactivation of both diseases. Biologic response modifiers are also contraindicated for those with a history of lymphoma and may result in severe allergic responses in some patients because they are derived from proteins and not chemicals.

13. 4. If a Navajo patient tells the nurse that he has "ghost sickness," the most appropriate response is: "How does ghost sickness make you feel?" This response respects the patient's perception of the disease and helps the nurse to understand what symptoms the patient is attributing to the disorder. The Navajo believe that ghost sickness is brought about by evil spirits and believe that a tribal healer may be able to overcome the spirit. Typical symptoms include weakness, nightmares, fear, and feelings of suffocation.

14. 2. Doppler ultrasound is used primarily to assess blood flow (direction, speed). As part of an abdominal ultrasound, Doppler ultrasound may help to identify impaired circulation to the organs as well as changes in blood flow associated with tumors. Doppler imaging differentiates between antegrade (expected forward movement) and retrograde (unexpected movement) blood flow. Doppler imaging is often used to assess hepatic blood flow as different disease processes result in distinctive changes in blood flow.

15. 3. If the nurse is using the BVMGR (beliefs, values, meanings, goals, and relationships) rubric for implementing spiritual care, these aspects apply to assessment of the patient. That is, the nurse should try to understand the patient's BVMGR and should not let personal BVMGR intrude and should avoid any indication of proselytizing when the nurse's BVMGR is at odds with the patient.

While the nurse may not share the patient's belief system, the nurse should always seek to understand and to show respect for it.

16. 1. Capsule endoscopy is used primarily to examine the small intestine, which, because of its length, is otherwise difficult to assess as it cannot be reached with colonoscopy or esophagogastroduodenoscopy. The capsule, which is swallowed by the patient, contains a miniature camera and LEDs. The camera wirelessly transmits pictures to a receiver as it passes through the small intestine. The capsule is usually passed anally within 24 to 48 hours although there is a small risk of retention.

17. 4. A history of diabetes mellitus, major abdominal/thoracic trauma, and neurological disorders increases the risk of aspiration for a patient receiving tube feedings. Patients should be positioned with the head elevated to 45 degrees if possible and supine position avoided. Continuous feedings pose less risk than intermittent or bolus feedings, and the older patient is at greater risk than the younger. Metoclopramide may be given to increase the rate of gastric emptying. The tube should be checked for correct position at every feeding or every 4 to 6 hours if feedings are continuous.

18. 3. If a patient complains of increasing abdominal pain and has been passing 3 to 4 sticky foul-smelling stools for 4 days, exhibits postural hypotension, and has a hemoglobin of is 9.2 mg/dL (92 mmol/L) and hematocrit 28%, the nurse should suspect iron deficiency anemia with upper GI bleeding. The anemia occurs from blood loss (low hemoglobin and hematocrit with normal MCV) and the melena is from blood in the upper GI tract that is exposed to digestive enzymes. The BUN is often elevated because of increased absorption of blood.

19. 2. If a patient has been prescribed antibiotic therapy and probiotics to help to maintain intestinal flora, the antibiotic and the probiotics at least 2 hours apart because the antibiotic can kill not only the bacteria already present in the intestines but also the bacteria in the probiotics. Probiotics that contain *Saccharomyces boulardii* also may help to reduce toxins produced by *Clostridium difficile*. Patients who are severely immunocompromised and taking long-term broad-spectrum antibiotics have developed sepsis from probiotics, so probiotics should be used with care in these patients.

20. 1. If the nurse hears a patient's physician complaining that a patient is "difficult and impatient," and the nurse tells the physician that the patient is very frightened and acting defensively, the aspect of care that the nurse is exhibiting is advocacy. The nurse is speaking up in defense of the patient and acting for the patient's benefit in trying to help the physician have a more balanced view of the patient's behavior.

21. 1. If imaging shows that a patient has an intestinal obstruction from a cancerous lesion at the duodenum, the signs and symptoms likely include copious emesis of undigested food (with no evidence of bile) after eating, succession splashing bowel sounds in the left upper quadrant but generally absence of abdominal pain or distention. If the condition persists untreated, the patient may show signs of dehydration and muscle wasting. The stomach may begin to dilate and excessive peristaltic action may be evident.

22. 2. The nurse should advise a patient to avoid taking St. John's wort when taking immunosuppressant drugs. St. John's wort is commonly used to treat depression and anxiety; however, it may interact with many different drugs, so if patients indicate an interest in taking the herbal preparation, the nurse should carefully review the patient's list of drugs. St. John's wort should also not be taken with antibiotics, birth control pills, antidepressants, warfarin, or anticonvulsants.

23. 3. If two grounding pads (AKA return electrodes) are utilized during a procedure involving electrical cautery, a correct placement is the right upper thigh and the left upper thigh. Grounding pads should be placed at a distance from the surgical site and, if two are utilized, they should be placed equidistantly and symmetrically and never on just one limb as this increases the risk of burns. Using two pads divides the current and reduces risk of burns. The pads must be fully in contact with the skin and placed according to manufacturer's directions.

24. 2. When reviewing medications for a patient with cirrhosis, the nurse must consider that the liver disease may affect drug metabolism, which is the process of biotransformation. While some metabolism occurs in the skeletal muscles, lungs, kidneys, plasma, and intestines, most metabolism occurs in the liver through the action of microsomal enzymes (AKA cytochrome P-450 enzymes). These enzymes target primarily lipophilic drugs, which comprise the majority of drugs in common use.

25. 4. Autonomy is the ethical principle that the individual has the right to make decisions about his/her own care, based on informed consent and understanding of risks and benefits. Beneficence is an ethical principle that involves performing actions that are for the purpose of benefitting another person. Nonmaleficence is an ethical principle that means healthcare workers should provide care in a manner that does not cause direct intentional harm to the patient. Justice is the ethical principle that relates to the distribution of the limited resources of healthcare benefits to the members of society.

26. 1. If a patient with inflammatory bowel disease (IBD) has bouts of severe diarrhea but is unsure of the cause, the nurse should advise the patient to maintain a food diary, writing down all food and fluid intake to see if a pattern emerges. While many patients with IBD are lactose intolerant, testing can show if this is the problem. Increasing fat or fiber in the diet may aggravate the diarrhea.

27. 4. Absorption of nutrients from the small bowel is often impaired in older adults because of broadening and shortening of villi, which decreases the surface area available. Additionally, levels of some enzymes decrease. For example, lactase levels may fall, and this can cause increased lactose intolerance. When fecal material moves slowly through the bowels, bacterial overgrowth may occur, and this can affect absorption of nutrients because the bacteria require nutrients and can also cause diarrhea, which interferes with absorption.

28. 2. If a 72-year-old patient has polyps removed, the type of polyp that is precancerous is the adenomatous polyp, which can include tubular adenomas, tubular villous adenoma, and villous adenoma. Polyps associated with hereditary polyposis syndromes (familial adenomatous polyposis) are also precancerous. Patients with precancerous polyps are generally advised to have routine follow-up colonoscopies every 3 years because of increased risk of colon cancer.

29. 3. The nurse is educating a patient who is to be discharged after surgery to remove a cancerous lesion of the colon and create a colostomy. The nurse advises the patient that some foods may cause:

- Odor: fish, eggs, onions, broccoli, asparagus, and cabbage.
- Gas: beans, carbonated beverages, strong cheeses, beer, and sprouts.
- Diarrhea: beer, green beans, coffee, raw fruits, spicy foods, and spinach.
- Obstruction: popcorn, seeds, raw vegetables, nuts, and corn.

30. 1. If, following a colonoscopy with removal of polyps, a patient developed abdominal pain with elevated temperature, WBC count, and C-reactive protein, the patient should have an abdominal CT

to differentiate between thermal injury causing perforation and one causing post-polypectomy electrocoagulation syndrome (transmural burn without perforation). Symptoms for both are similar initially, but post-polypectomy electrocoagulation syndrome heals with conservative treatment while perforation requires surgical repair.

31. 4. If a patient develops an infection with a multi-drug resistant organism (MDRO), the nurse anticipates that the patient's history will show previous antibiotic use as this is a factor in almost all cases. Other risk factors include prolonged hospitalization and intraabdominal surgery. MDRO infections are increasingly resistant to 2 or more antibiotics, including vancomycin. Restriction of vancomycin use alone has not proven successful in controlling development of MDRO because multiple other antibiotics are implicated.

32. 3. The standard triple therapy for *H. pylori*-associated peptic ulcer disease include a proton pump inhibitor BID, clarithromycin 500 mg BID, and amoxicillin 1 g BID. Metronidazole 500 mg BID may be substituted for amoxicillin for those with penicillin allergy. Treatment is usually continued for 10 to 14 days. Using two antibiotics is especially important because of increasing resistant strains. The standard triple therapy is most commonly utilized, but a standard quadruple therapy and sequential quadruple therapy may also be considered.

33. 1. When lifting an item, the muscles in the legs should be used. The nurse should stand close to the item or person being lifted and use the leg muscles to support weight rather than the arms or back and should stoop down rather than bending over. If items or people are heavy, then lift devices should be used rather than lifting manually. If items are up high, the nurse should avoid stretching but should use a step stool or gripping device to reach the item.

34. 2. When palpating a patient's abdomen, a positive Murphy's sign (sudden holding of breath with RUQ palpation) indicates cholecystitis. Murphy's sign is usually negative with choledocholithiasis although cholecystitis is most often caused by gallstones that obstruct the flow of bile, causing the gallbladder to swell and become inflamed. However, cholecystitis may also result from tumors or impaired circulation (common with diabetics). Typical symptoms include nausea and vomiting and severe middle or RUQ abdominal pain.

35. 3. If a patient is receiving methotrexate for maintenance treatment of Crohn's disease, laboratory tests that should be routinely monitored include the CBC and renal (creatinine and BUN) and liver function tests. FDA guidelines advise testing at least every 1 to 2 months during therapy, but some authorities recommend testing every 2 to 4 weeks during the first few months of treatment. Adverse effects of methotrexate include renal failure, portal fibrosis, myelosuppression, headache, and rash.

36. 2. If a patient presents with symptoms consistent with diverticulosis, the imaging technique that will likely be used to confirm the diagnosis is colonoscopy, which allows biopsy to rule out other disorders and allows visualization of involvement. Ultrasound shows non-specific abnormalities and cannot conclusively diagnose diverticulitis, colonic contrast studies, such as barium enema, have limited value because most diverticula are extraluminal, and it increases the risk of perforation if peritoneal irritation is present.

37. 1. The primary tests that screen for hepatitis include alanine transaminase (ALT) (normal 5-35 units) and aspartate transaminase (AST) (normal 10-40 units). These are liver enzymes that increase with inflammation and damage to hepatic cells. ALT is more specific than AST and usually shows a higher increase. ALT may increase to 10 times normal with acute infection and 2 to 3 times

normal with chronic infection, so ALT is used most often to monitor treatment. However, many drugs can affect ALT results, so medication reconciliation is essential.

38. 4. Healthcare-associated infections kill almost 100,000 people each year in the United States, and environmental contamination is a factor in 20% to 40% of HAIs, with pathogens carried from environmental surfaces on the hands of healthcare workers. Pathogens that are of increasing concern are norovirus, *Clostridium difficile*, *Acinetobacter* species, MR*SA* and vancomycin-resistant *Enterococcus.* Patients admitted to rooms previously occupied by patients infected with these pathogens are at increased risk because the agents are capable of surviving for prolonged periods in the environment.

39. 3. The Spaulding system of sterilization and disinfection:

- **Critical:** Contact sterile tissue or the vascular system, including surgical instruments, IV catheters, and prosthetic implants. Contamination poses a high risk of infection, so these items must be sterile.
- **Semi-critical:** Contact mucous membranes or non-intact skin, including endoscopes, diaphragm fitting rings, and laryngoscope blades. These tissues tend to be more resistant to spores, so these items can be disinfected with high-level disinfectants.
- **Non-critical:** Contact intact skin only, including patient care items such as blood pressure cuffs and bedpans and environmental surfaces. Decontamination can be done at point of care.

40. 2. If, following removal of the esophagogastroduodenoscopy tube, the patient begins to cough violently and appears cyanotic, the most appropriate initial intervention is to suction the airway and increase supplemental oxygen. These symptoms are consistent with aspiration of gastric fluids, which can lead to aspiration pneumonia. The patient needs an x-ray and antibiotic therapy. Patients with gastric bleeding, gastric obstruction, excessive sedation, and older adults are especially at risk of aspiration during endoscopic procedures.

41. 3. The CDC recommended method of routine hand hygiene is now using alcohol-based hand rubs. This can be done relatively quickly, and compliance tends to be better than washing hands with soap and water. However, if the hands are visibly soiled or have come into contact with bodily fluids, then they must be thoroughly washed with soap and water to remove all residue. Additionally, if the healthcare provider is exposed to spore-producing microbes, such as *B. anthracis* or *C. difficile,* or norovirus, then washing with soap and water is required.

42. 4. In regards to reprocessing of single-use devices, the CMS recommends use of third-party reprocessors because of the stringency of the regulations by the FDA for reprocessing and the type of equipment needed. The trend is toward increased reprocessing of single-use devices because of the costs of medical care. The FDA categorizes medical devices as class I, II, or III with class I posting the lowest risk to the patient and class III the highest. Requirements for reprocessing of class III devices are more stringent than for class I or II.

43. 2. The incubation period for foodborne illness caused by *Salmonella* spp. is one to three days, and the infection persists for four to seven days. Symptoms include fever, abdominal cramping, and diarrhea. *S. typhi* and *S. paratyphi* result in more severe symptoms and typhoid fever. Infection often results from contaminated poultry, eggs, unpasteurized milk products or juices, and raw fruits and vegetables. Outbreaks may occur if the water supply becomes contaminated. Antibiotics are usually contraindicated except for *S. typhi* and *S paratyphi.*

44. 3. Constipation is usually defined as fewer than three stools per week although there is considerable individual variation. Some people have two to three stools daily while others only defecate every two or three days, so it's necessary to determine the normal pattern for a patient when assessing constipation. Constipation is also sometimes described in terms of stool consistency (hard, small) and difficulty defecating (need to strain, splinting). Constipation is most common in patients in their 60's, with rates about 5 times those of younger adults.

45. 4. **Bowel retraining** strategies include:

- Keeping a bowel diary for a week.
- Modifying diet and fluid intake to assure normal stool consistency, including increased fiber and fluids, eating meals at scheduled times, and avoiding foods that increase bowel dysfunction.
- Establishing a schedule for defecation, preferably at the same time each day and about 20-30 minutes after a meal.
- Practicing Kegel exercises.
- Using a stimulus to promote defecation, such as enemas, suppositories, or laxatives in the beginning, with a goal to decrease such use. Digital stimulation or hot drinks may be used.
- Keeping a record of stool consistency and evacuation.

46. 1. If a patient is receiving enteral feeding, administration of cold formula is most likely to contribute to diarrhea. Other causes of diarrhea include rapid infusion and bolus feedings, and hyperosmolar formula. If diarrhea occurs, the patient's feedings should be re-evaluated (rate slowed, change in formula) and fluid balance and electrolyte status assessed. Medications should be assessed and pro-motility medications avoided as they may contribute to diarrhea.

47. 4. For the bowel transit time test, patients take capsules that contain radiopaque markers and then continue with their regular diet. They return 5 days later for radiographs. Typically, about 80% of the markers are excreted in 5 days, so if fewer than 20% remain, then transit time is faster than normal and more than 20%, slower than normal. This test results are affected by the types of foods and amount of liquids consumed, so results must be evaluated in terms of diet and other factors.

48. 3. If a patient has developed acne, weight gain, mood swings, and hyperglycemia, the most likely cause is prednisone, a corticosteroid. Corticosteroids are prescribed to suppress the immune response and reduce inflammation, but have numerous adverse effects so they are usually used for short periods rather than extended use. Other possible adverse effects include insomnia, hypertension, osteoporosis, moon facies, glaucoma, cataracts, and increased risk of infection.

49. 1. Omeprazole (Prilosec®), a proton pump inhibitor, suppresses secretion of gastric acids and is used primarily to treat GERD and erosive esophagitis. Omeprazole should be taken on an empty stomach to be most effective. Adverse effects include stomach pain, nausea and vomiting, diarrhea, flatulence, and headache. In rare cases, patients may develop severe myopathy. Drug interactions may occur with methotrexate, clopidogrel, and St. John's wort.

50. 2. While all of these are important factors in fecal incontinence, the most common cause is fecal impaction, which may result from chronic constipation. Chronic constipation increases pressure on the anal sphincters and can damage nerves and muscles. Additionally, transit time through the large intestine is often slowed with constipation, increasing fluid absorption and contributing to impaction. When stool becomes impacted, the body compensates by increasing fluid in the stool

above the impaction, resulting in diarrhea stool leaking about the impaction and through the damaged sphincters.

51. 4. The Bristol Stool Form has descriptions and pictures to help people identify the correct type of stool.

Type 1: Separate small hard lumps of stool that are difficult to pass.
Type 2: Sausage-shaped lumpy stool.
Type 3: Sausage-shaped and lumpy but with cracks on the surface.
Type 4: Long, smooth, soft, snake-like stool.
Type 5: Soft blobs of stool that are easily passed and have clear-cut edges.
Type 6: Mushy, fluffy pieces of stool with uneven ragged edges.
Type 7: Watery stool that is entirely liquid.

The bowel diary should include the time of each event (defecation, incontinence, and flatus), type of stool, amount, activity at the time of incontinence, intake of food and drinks, and all medications.

52. 1. If a patient has been dieting but complains that she has developed chronic diarrhea, the item on the food log that is most likely the cause is dietetic hard candy. Dietetic candy, diet soda, sugarless gum, and other sugarless products contain sweeteners (such as sorbitol, sucralose, and xylitol) that often cause diarrhea, abdominal distention, and gas, especially if taken in large amounts. The patient should stop eating the dietetic candy until the diarrhea stops and then eat in only small amounts to tolerance.

53. 3. If a patient has prescriptions from four different doctors and admits to taking additional "pills" but can't recall which ones and gives conflicting information regarding the dosage and frequency of the different medications, the nurse should recognize these findings as an indication of polypharmacy. Polypharmacy occurs when patients take too many drugs, some of which may be duplicates or may interact with other drugs, especially when prescriptions are from multiple physicians.

54. 2. The most common cause of upper GI bleeding is peptic ulcer disease (about 50%) while the most common cause of lower GI bleeding is diverticulosis (about 50%). Symptoms of upper GI bleeding include epigastric pain and hematemesis. Melena may occur with both upper and lower GI bleeding but is most common with upper GI. Treatment varies depending on the cause, but those who are hemodynamically unstable require immediate resuscitation to maintain adequate blood pressure while the patient is being typed and cross-matched for transfusions.

55. 3. When teaching a patient to care for a PEG feeding tube, the gerontological nurse should tell the patient that, in order to prevent dumping syndrome, the patient should stay in semi-Fowler's position for one hour after feedings as this slows transit time by decreasing the force of gravity. Additionally, formula should be instilled slowly and at room temperature and small volumes of water used to flush the tubing before and after feedings because diluted formula has a faster transit time. Continuous drip also results in less incidence of dumping syndrome than bolus administration.

56. 1. The Health Insurance Portability and Accountability Act (HIPPA) addresses the rights of the individual related to privacy of health information. The nurse must not release any information or documentation about a patient's condition or treatment without consent, as the individual has the right to determine who has access to personal information, which is considered protected health information (PHI), including health history, condition, treatments in any form, and any

documentation. Personal information can be shared with spouse, legal guardians, and those with durable power of attorney.

57. 2. If a 69-year-old patient is learning to care for a colostomy but is quite tense and becomes confused about the sequence of actions required, the most appropriate teaching strategy is to breaks the tasks into small steps and teach sequentially. When the patient becomes adept at one step, the patient can begin to learn the next. When patients are ill and stressed, learning can be difficult; and procedures, such as colostomy care, can seem overwhelming.

58. 4. These symptoms are consistent with a duodenal ulcer, and the positive urea breath test indicates a *Helicobacter pylori* infection, which is usually treated with a proton pump inhibitor plus clarithromycin and amoxicillin/metronidazole. About 90% of duodenal ulcers are associated with *H.pylori* infection. *H.pylori* weakens the mucosa and results in hypersecretion of gastric acid. Eating may increase pain with gastric ulcers but usually relieves pain with duodenal ulcers. Smoking increases the risk of peptic ulcer disease, and use of NSAIDs increases risk of serious complications, such as bleeding or perforation.

59. 3. Every 10 years. Screening should begin at age 50 or those with average risk and age 40 with increased risk. Screening tests include:

- Colonoscopy—every 10 years or as follow-up for abnormalities in other screening: Allows for removal of polyps, small cancerous lesions, and biopsies and provides surveillance of inflammatory bowel disease.
- Fecal occult blood—yearly: checks for blood in stool.
- Flexible sigmoidoscopy—every 5 years: Scope checks for polyps or signs of cancer in rectum and lower third of colon.
- Double contrast barium enema—every 5 years: X-ray with contrast to visualize intestinal abnormalities.

60. 2. Miller-Abbott is a long double-lumen tube inserted into the small intestine for drainage and decompression. The Salem-sump tube is also double-lumen but is short and contains a small vent tube within the larger tube to help reduce pressure at the distal eyes to less than 24 mm Hg in order to prevent tissue damage. The Cantor tube is a single lumen tube that contains an inflatable balloon at the distal end to prevent the tube from migrating. The Levin tube is a single lumen tube with a solid end.

61. 2. The electrolyte imbalance that is likely to occur with persistent vomiting and diarrhea is hyponatremia. Gastric and intestinal fluids contain high levels of sodium, so sodium can become depleted with nausea and diarrhea. Hyponatremia is a sodium level of less than 135 mEq/L. This type of hyponatremia resulting from hypovolemia is characterized by dry mucous membranes, orthostatic hypotension, tachycardia and poor skin turgor. The patient may appear weak, stuporous, confused and/or lethargic.

62. 3. Most absorption of nutrients occurs in the small intestine, in the jejunum and ileum. The digestive process starts in the mouth as saliva and chewing begin to break down the food that then enters the esophagus and travels to the stomach, where the food is further mixed and broken down by the addition of acid and enzymes. This process continues in the duodenum with most absorption of nutrients occurring in the small intestine. Fluid continues to be absorbed in the large intestine.

63. 4. Bulk-forming products, such as psyllium (Metamucil®), methycellulose (Citrucel®) and polycarbophil (Fibercon®) are generally the drugs of choice for chronic constipation because they

increase absorption of fluid in the stool, helping to increase mass, soften stool, and stimulate peristalsis. Bulk-forming products have few adverse effects and are less irritating to the intestines than other preparations. However, if fluid intake is inadequate, bulk formers can cause obstruction, so they should be avoided with patients who are dehydrated or on fluid restriction.

64. 2. The tract of a PEG usually matures and heals within 2 to 4 weeks. Once the tract has healed, the original PEG tube can generally be replaced with a balloon gastrostomy tube. Gastrostomy tubes with an internal balloon or mushroom tip, measured markings, and an external disk are easier to stabilize, but internal devices should be checked daily by gently pulling until resistance is felt. External stabilizing devices can be applied to the skin to hold the tube in place. The tube may also be taped to the abdomen or secured with a binder.

65. 1. While the stoma may be edematous in the initial postoperative period, it should appear red to pink, shiny, and moist, indicating adequate oxygenation and healthy tissue. If the stoma appears dull and cyanotic (blue to purple to brown/black if the tissue becomes necrotic), the physician should be notified immediately because reoperation to increase blood flow to the tissue may be indicated. The stoma should be assessed for circulatory impairment on a regular schedule after surgery.

66. 4. The Kock pouch may need to be irrigated postoperatively to promote drainage because of the accumulation of mucus. Also, once the patient begins to eat, drainage may slow, requiring irrigation. Up to 1000 mL total of solution (usually tap water) may be needed to flush the pouch but only 30 to 40 mL of fluid should be instilled at one time as the capacity of the pouch is small. The instilled fluid should be drained completely before doing another instillation and the patient observed carefully for abdominal discomfort.

67. 3. Unpreserved stool must be tested for ova and parasites within 2 hours of collection. (The same is true for most tests with unpreserved stool.) However, the stool may be place in liquid transport media with preservative, such as orange Cary-Blair container, and tested within 14 days for ova and parasites or cultured. WBC count must be carried out on unpreserved stool. Testing for rotavirus must also be carried out on unpreserved stool immediately after collection.

68. 2. Increased frequency of stools, bloody diarrhea, fever, and fecal incontinence are signs of pouchitis, non-specific inflammation of the pouch. Although the cause is not known, pouchitis may indicate undiagnosed regional enteritis (Crohn's disease) in some patients although it is more common in patients with ulcerative colitis. Pouchitis is most common in the first two years after surgery. Pouchitis usually responds rapidly to metronidazole, and this helps to differentiate the condition from others that may cause similar symptoms.

69. 4. The pH of gastric fluids is usually 0 to 4, so this finding may indicate proximal migration of the J-tube. The pH in the small intestine is usually less than 6 while a higher pH, such as >7.5 may indicate pulmonary migration. A marked increase in intestinal residual volume may indicate migration. If that occurs, then feedings should be held for at least an hour before pH testing is done. Gastric aspirant is usually curdled and clear to white while intestinal aspirant may be brownish/greenish because of bile staining.

70. 1. The initial goal of enterocutaneous fistula management is to control fluid and electrolyte imbalance. Dehydration is frequent with high-output fistulae, and patients may develop hyponatremia and hypokalemia with metabolic acidosis. Parenteral nutrition, if necessary, should be initiated after the fluid/electrolyte balance is re-established. Up to 90% of patients with enterocutaneous fistulae develop malnutrition, and if patients are unable to obtain adequate

nutrition orally, then enteral or parenteral feedings may be indicated, depending on the site of the fistula.

71. 4. The complication that is most common outside of the gastrointestinal tract with patients with inflammatory bowel disease is anemia. Patient's often have poor nutritional status with inadequate protein and iron in their diets and may have blood loss associated with lesions. Osteoporosis is also a common finding, and some patients have experienced other disorders, such as interstitial cystitis, fibromyalgia, and migraines. Those with Crohn's disease often have inflammation of joints and eyes.

72. 1. The external fixation device of a PEG tube should be placed 1 to 2 cm above the skin surface to prevent excessive tension that may result in buried bumper syndrome in which the internal fixation device becomes lodged in the mucosal lining of the gastric wall, resulting in ulceration. Rotating the PEG tube also helps to prevent BBS. Typical symptoms of BBS include increasing abdominal pain and difficulty infusing the feeding solution. If BBS occurs, the PEG must be replaced.

73. 2. Insertion of balloon replacement gastrostomy tube:

1. Gather supplies, position patient to 30°.
2. Inject 20 ml sterile water into balloon port to check leaks; withdraw water and retain filled syringe.
3. Move external disk to near distal end and catheter tip.
4. Cleanse peristomal area with NS in spiral movement. Dry skin.
5. Insert tube gently to pre-measured distance and inflate balloon.
6. Gently pull tube until resistance met. Slide external bumper to 1.5cm from skin surface.
7. Rotate tube in circular motion to ensure free rotation.
8. Use 30-60 ml syringe to aspirate gastric content. Flush tube with water.
9. Apply barriers and mark exit measurement.

74. 3. A Durable Power of Attorney is the legal document that designates someone to make decisions regarding medical and end-of-life care if a patient is mentally incompetent. This is a type of Advance Directive, which can include living wills or specific requests of the patient regarding treatment. A Do-Not-Resuscitate order indicates the patient does not want resuscitative treatment for terminal illness or condition. A General Power of Attorney allows a designated person to make decisions for a person over broader areas, including financial.

75. 1. If a 30-year-old patient with Crohn's disease is disabled and uninsured because of illness but unable to afford medications to control the disease, the most likely source of financial assistance is Medicaid. Medicaid is a joint program of the federal and states governments, so eligibility criteria may vary from state to state, but Medicaid provides medical benefits, including the costs of drugs, to people with low income. People with disabilities, which can include Crohn's disease, are in one of the categories eligible to apply for Medicaid.

76. 3. With cardiac arrest, immediate defibrillation is indicated for ventricular fibrillation and ventricular tachycardia (VF/VT) but is not indicated for pulseless electrical activity (PEA) or asystole because these conditions do not respond. Adrenaline (Epinephrine) (IV 1 mg) and vasopressin (40 units) may be repeatedly administered with PEA, asystole, or VF and when two shocks have been unsuccessful. For VF/VT immediate defibrillation should be carried out, followed by CPR for 2 minutes and repeat defibrillation if necessary.

77. 2. If a patient is scheduled the next day for an abdominal ultrasound to evaluate the liver, pancreas, and bile ducts, the nurse anticipates that the patient will be advised to have a fat-free

dinner the evening before and be NPO after midnight. Ultrasound is a non-invasive technique that utilizes high-frequency sound waves to create images (size, shape, contours, consistency) of internal structures. These images are viewed on a monitor during the procedure.

78. 4. If a 70-year-old patient has advanced gastric carcinoma, the criteria that makes the patient eligible for Hospice care is if the patient has stopped curative treatments and life expectancy is 6 months or less. Patients under hospice care are allowed palliative treatment to relieve pain, nausea, and other discomforts. Disease-specific requirements include AIDS, cancer, liver disease, dementia, kidney disease, cardiac disease, stroke, and neurological disorders. Hospice benefits include medications (to control symptoms), medical equipment, nursing assessment, respite care (up to 5 days), and part-time aides.

79. 3. The most common site for obstruction of the small intestine is the ileum, usually associated with adhesions (70%) with the rest caused by hernias, IBS (which can result in strictures), or malignancies. Over 90% of patients who undergo abdominal surgery eventually develop adhesions. Obstructions of the colon are more likely to be associated with malignancies (60%). Diagnosis of small bowel obstruction is based on physical examination and symptoms and is typically confirmed with abdominal x-ray and/or CT scan.

80. 1. If a patient who has undergone cholecystectomy develops paralytic ileus, the most likely intervention is insertion of an NG tube and decompression. Antibiotics are generally not indicated. If the patient has been receiving enteral feedings, they should be discontinued. IV resuscitation is indicated while the NG tube is in place and replacement of electrolytes as needed (especially potassium). Diagnosis is usually confirmed with x-ray and/or CT scan and to rule out mechanical obstruction, which requires surgical intervention.

81. 4. The acid-base disorder that is most common with acute mesenteric ischemia is metabolic acidosis. Other laboratory findings include increased WBC count, lactate, and amylase. Presenting symptoms usually include both abdominal pain and melena. Mesenteric ischemia, which can be caused by arterial hypoperfusion, impaired drainage of venous blood, or thrombosis, results in ischemia of the bowel and mild to severe damage of the tissue. In some cases, bowel ischemia can result from non-occlusive causes, such as impaired cardiac output (heart failure, cardiac arrest). In cases associated with occlusive causes, surgical repair is needed.

82. 2. If bacteria, such as *Escherichia coli*, produce extended spectrum beta lactamase (ESBL), the nurse should anticipate that the bacteria will be resistant to multiple antibiotics. The enzymes produced are able to destroy active ingredients found in antibiotics, such as cephalosporins and beta lactamases. ESBLs were first detected in the 1960s in Greece and in 1988 in the US. ESBLs have been associated with diarrhea, skin infections, pneumonia, UTIs, and sepsis. Most ESBL-bacteria respond to carbapenems at present although CREs pose an increasing threat.

83. 1. The form of anesthesia that is most commonly used when a patient requires removal of a foreign object from the rectum is a benzodiazepine to relax the patient and an opioid for pain control. Objects can generally be removed in the ED if they are within 10 cm of anus and palpable by digital exam. Patients are usually placed in the lithotomy position. An anal or vaginal speculum may be needed to facilitate removal. If an object cannot be safely removed, surgical intervention may be needed.

84. 3. The most common positioning for a patient who is to undergo a rigid sigmoidoscopy for sigmoid volvulus or other purpose is the left lateral (Sims) position. The patient's hips should slightly extend beyond the edge of the table, and the patient's knees should be flexed. A small

sandbag is often placed under the left hip. Rigid sigmoidoscopy is usually carried out with sedation, but must be preceded by a digital rectal exam. Rigid sigmoidoscopy is contraindicated with anal stenosis or bowel perforation.

85. 2. If a patient has received midazolam for an endoscopic procedure, the peak effect occurs within 3 to 5 minutes with duration of 1 to 3 hours. Romazicon (Flumazenil®) may be administered as a reversal agent. The narcotic usually administered with midazolam is fentanyl with peak effect occurring within 5 to 8 minutes and the same 1- to 3-hour duration. Naloxone (Narcan®) may be administered as a reversal agent.

86. 1. If a patient is to receive antibiotic prophylaxis for placement of PEG tube, the antibiotic should be administered 30 minutes before the procedure begins. All patients who are to have PEG placement should receive antibiotic prophylaxis. The most commonly administered prophylaxis is ampicillin (2 g) and gentamicin (1.5 mg/kg) unless the patient has an allergy to penicillin. In that case, vancomycin (1 g) may be administered as an alternative.

87. 2. According to Health.gov recommendations for fiber intake, 14 grams of fiber should be consumed for each 1000 calories. High fiber foods include beans, lentils, fruit, Brussels sprouts, spinach, corn, sweet potatoes, and whole grain breads and cereals. Some fiber (soluble) dissolves into a viscous gel and other fiber (insoluble) acts like a sponge and soaks up water. Fiber helps to slow gastric emptying, promote a sense of fullness, increase bulk in the stool, and prevent constipation.

88. 1. If, within 90 seconds of receiving midazolam for an endoscopic procedure, the patient exhibits signs of anaphylaxis with bronchospasm and severe hypotension, the correct initial emergent response is to administer epinephrine. The usual SQ/IM dosage is 0.1% (1:1000) and IV dosage is 0.01% (1:10,000). If administered IM, the vastus lateralis muscle of the thigh is the preferred site. Additional medications include albuterol (inhaled), antihistamine (diphenhydramine), corticosteroid, and H-1 an H-2 blockers (ranitidine).

89. 4. A stool specimen to test for *Clostridium difficile* may be held for 24 hours at room temperature or 5 days under refrigeration at 2° to 8° C. The specimen must remain unpreserved and needs to be very soft, liquid or semi-liquid. Testing cannot be carried out if the stool is hard or formed because the amount of toxin present in the stool is minimal. Additionally, if the patient is infected with *C. difficile,* the patient likely has 3 or more liquid stools daily.

90. 3. The esophageal pH probe is usually let in place for 24 hours. It is inserted nasally and attached to a monitor that continually assesses acidity. In some cases, a 48-hour probe is used. This 48-hour probe has a small monitor attached to a catheter and placed at the distal portion of the esophagus. It sends acidity recordings wirelessly to a recorder worn on the body and automatically detaches and passes through the intestinal tract after 48 hours.

91. 4. Once a rubber band ligation is carried out for a second-degree hemorrhoid, the tissue usually sloughs off within about 7 to 14 days. The band is placed about the base of the hemorrhoid, effectively cutting off circulation to the hemorrhoid. Most people experience mild pain/discomfort and may have slight bleeding. However, a small risk of severe bleeding and sepsis exists. Patients should be advised to increase fiber to prevent constipation and to take a Sitz bath after defecation.

92. 1. If using the FAITH mnemonic as a guide to spiritual assessment, the H stands for Help:

F	Is there a **faith**, religion, or spiritual belief important to you?
A	How does your belief system **apply** to your health?
I	What **involvement** do you have in a church or faith community?
T	Is your **treatment** affected by your spiritual beliefs?
H	What **help** can I give you with spiritual concerns?

93. 3. The most common reason for sexual dysfunction after an ileostomy/colostomy is psychological inhibitions. The patient may fear rejection, odor, or spillage and may be unsure of how to broach the subject of the ileostomy/colostomy with a partner. Some patients find coping with the change in body image difficult. Patients often benefit from participating in a support group and from guidance in sexual matters. For example, patients may feel more comfortable wearing undergarments (boxer shorts, crotchless panties) during sexual activity.

94. 2. Patients who have had bariatric surgery should generally limit total meal size to less than one cup and should eat 3 meals daily and 2 snacks of protein. The patient should avoid drinking liquids for 15 minutes before meals and 90 minutes after and should avoid liquids that contain calories (sodas, juices, wine/beer). Food choices should be high in nutrition. Patients should be advised to be aware of thirst and to observe urine for signs of dehydration.

95. 3. If administering a bolus feeding of 400 mL per a gastrostomy tube, the feeding should generally be given over 10 to 15 minutes per gravity (raising and lowering the container to control flow). The patient's response can help to guide administration. If the patient feels suddenly full, the rate should be slowed. Intermittent feedings are usually administered on a regular schedule for about 30 minutes at a time.

96. 1. If, following gastric surgery with removal of the pylorus, a patient develops bile reflux gastritis/esophagitis, the treatment that is most indicated is cholestyramine (Questran®). Cholestyramine binds bile acids in the intestines and causes them to be excreted in the feces. Cholestyramine may decrease absorption of numerous drugs/substances (including beta blockers, corticosteroid, fat-soluble vitamins, thiazides, penicillin, and thyroid hormones), so these drugs must be administered 1 hour prior to cholestyramine or 4 hours after.

97. 4. Diarrhea:

Type	Cause
Exudative	Radiation and chemotherapy
Infectious	Infectious agents, such as *Clostridium difficile*
Malabsorptive	Decreased serum albumin
Osmotic	Intestinal hemorrhage, pancreatic impairment, and lactose intolerance
Secretory	Bacterial toxins and neoplasms

98. 2. In order to prevent *Escherichia coli* infection from eating contaminated meat, all ground beef should be cooked to at least 160° F, and the temperature should be verified by thermometer as appearance may vary. Raw meats should always be kept separate from other foods, and dairy products and juices should be pasteurized. Fruits and vegetables should be washed under clean running water. Alfalfa sprouts can harbor *E. coli*, so children under 5, older adults, and patients who are immunocompromised should avoid eating them.

99. 4. After the cuff of the Flexi-seal Fecal Management System® is inserted into the rectum, the nurse should use a syringe to fill the cuff with 45 mL water. Procedure:

1. Don PPI, place patient in left lateral knee-chest position, and connect catheter to the bag.
2. Withdraw air from cuff with syringe.
3. Flatten cuff and fold in half, lubricate.
4. Insert cuff into rectum and fill cuff with 45 mL water with syringe to inflate the balloon end of the cuff.
5. Gently tug the cuff into position to seal the rectum.

100. 1. The complication that is most likely to occur with ulcerative colitis is abscess. Abscesses form as the tissue ulcerates and becomes inflamed; however, because the disorder involves the superficial mucosa and is not transmural, fistulas, fissures, and obstructions (common with Crohn's disease) usually do not occur. Inflammation generally begins in the rectum and spreads proximally throughout the colon. Patients tend to experience periods of remission and exacerbation, and symptoms may be mild, severe, or fulminant.

101. 3. Patients with celiac disease must be advised to avoid food that contain gluten, which is a protein that is found in various grains, such as rye, barley, and wheat. Patients should eat oat products only if they are labeled as gluten-free because they may be contaminated by wheat products during processing in some facilities. Many processed foods and liquids (such as soups, beer, candy, processed meats) contain hidden gluten. Additionally, some medications utilize gluten-containing binding agents.

102. 4. The ethnic groups with the highest prevalence of ulcerative colitis are Caucasians and Ashkenazi (European) Jews. While the cause of ulcerative colitis is not clear, a genetic predisposition appears to play a role as family history is a risk factor. Studies have shown that patients with inflammatory bowel disease, such as ulcerative colitis and Crohn's disease, are also at increased risk of developing autoimmune disorders, such as multiple sclerosis and arthritis.

103. 3. If a 40-year-old patient with a history of Chagas disease reports increasing dysphagia, cough, regurgitation, drooling, and heartburn, the most likely cause is megaesophagus, resulting from destruction of neurons. Patients usually exhibit symptoms between ages 20 and 40 and may also have hypertrophy of the salivary glands, resulting in drooling because of excess saliva. Patients may also develop megacolon, which can lead to fecal impaction and bowel obstruction because of lack of motility.

104. 1. The drug of choice to treat *Giardia* infection is metronidazole (250 mg TID for 5 to 7 days). *Giardia* often contaminates water sources and spreads easily from person to person through fecal contact. Symptoms include abdominal pain/cramping, diarrhea (greasy stools), nausea, and vomiting. Patients often experience weight loss and have persistent symptoms for up to 3 weeks, and some people develop a chronic form of infection that can last for months or years.

105. 2. The most common test for pinworms is the cellophane test in which tape is touched to the perineal area several times and then examined under a microscope for eggs. This test has sensitivity of about 90%. The test should be done for 3 days in a row and when the patient first awakens in the morning. Stool specimens are usually negative because only about 5% of those infected have eggs in the stool.

106. 4. For moderate sedation (AKA conscious sedation) ASA guidelines require monitoring of capnography and pulse oximetry. Level of consciousness should be assessed at least every 5 minutes and supplemental oxygen provided unless otherwise contraindicated. Resuscitative

equipment and reversal agents (flumazenil and naloxone) must be available and a person trained in assessment and use available. During the recovery period after the procedure oxygenation, ventilation, and circulation should be monitored every 5 to 15 minutes.

107. 3. The primary reason for liver transplants is hepatitis C, which markedly increases risk of liver failure and hepatic cancer. Hepatitis C is spread through contact with blood or items contaminated with blood (shared needles, improperly sterilized equipment) and through sexual contact, tattooing, and piercing. No vaccine is available but antiviral treatments are available and up to 90% effective. Those with hepatitis C must avoid use of alcohol as it may cause progression of the disease.

108. 1. The most common carbapenem-resistant Enterobacteriaceae (CRE) in the United states is *Klebsiella pneumoniae* carbapenemase (KPC). New Delhi Metallo-beta-lactamase (NDM-1) is found in Pakistan and India. *Escherichia coli* carbapenemase (ECC), an increasing concern, is found in the Middle East, South American, India, and Southeast Asia. Verona Integron-Mediated Metallo-beta-lactamase (VIM) is found in Southern Europe, Southeast Asia, and scattered cases (Indiana) in the US.

109. 4. When examining the abdomen for bowel sounds, the nurse should auscultate for five minutes before determining that bowel sounds are absent. Most commonly, bowel sounds are heard 5 to 30 times a minute, usually heard best in the RLQ. Abnormal bowel sounds are classified as hyperactive (loud, high-pitched, gurgling), hypoactive (diminished), or absent (silent). Hyperactive sounds are associated with mechanical bowel obstruction (early), diarrhea, gastroenteritis, and use of laxatives. Hypoactive sounds are associated with peritonitis, and paralytic ileus, and late obstruction.

110. 2. If a patient who has recently had formation of an ileostomy suffers from disturbed body image, the best nursing intervention is to encourage the patient to verbalize feelings. The nurse must remain supportive and allow the patient to progress at his/her own speed in viewing and learning to care for the ileostomy. Some patients may benefit from counseling if their body image issues do not resolve or if they worsen.

111. 1. H2 blockers, such as cimetidine (Tagamet®), may decrease libido and increase erectile dysfunction, especially if taken in high doses or frequently during the day. These adverse effects tend to be worse with cimetidine than with other H2 blockers, so the patient may benefit from switching to a different drug or adjusting dosage. The nurse should question the patient about frequency of use and dosage of the drug and encourage the patient to discuss these issues with the physician.

112. 3 Glutaraldehyde 2%, hydrogen peroxide 7.5%, ortho-phthalaldehyde (OPA), as well as various hydrogen peroxide/peracetic acid combinations can provide high-level disinfection with 12 to 30 minutes of exposure. Manufacturer's recommendations for dilution and use must be followed carefully. Isopropyl and ethyl alcohol (70 to 90%), iodophor germicidal detergent, and sodium hypochlorite 5.25 to 6.15% can be used for intermediate and low-level disinfection at greater than 1-minute exposure.

113. 4. The primary treatment for norovirus infection is supportive care and fluids. Symptoms generally include diarrhea and vomiting with symptoms persisting for 1 to 3 days. Most people do not require treatment, but if diarrhea or vomiting is severe, an antiemetic or antidiarrheal may be prescribed if the patient is younger than 65. If severe dehydration occurs, the patient may require intravenous fluids until able to resume adequate oral intake.

114. 1. Almost all nutrients are absorbed by the small intestines, with the majority absorbed in the jejunum although some nutrients are absorbed at different parts of the small intestine:

- Jejunum: Sodium, chloride, fats, proteins, and carbohydrates.
- Ileum: Bile salts and vitamin B-12.
- Duodenum: Iron.
- Throughout the small bowel: Magnesium phosphate, water, lipids, and potassium.

Following a meal, residual wastes travel through the gastrointestinal tract and reach the terminal ileum within about 4 hours. Once in the large intestine, fluid and electrolytes continue to be absorbed and the stool thickens.

115. 3. While all foods can cause dyspepsia/indigestion, fatty foods usually cause the greatest discomfort because they are digested more slowly and stay in the stomach for a longer period of time. Patients with chronic dyspepsia may benefit from a low-fat diet. Some foods (spicy food, lettuce, gas-producing vegetables) may also result in increased discomfort. About a fourth of adults experience some degree of dyspepsia, which may include heartburn, bloating, feeling of fullness, and belching.

116. 4. If assisting with an endoscopic procedure, the nurse should expect to wear full surgical attire (gown, gloves, face mask, eye guard or face shield, hair and foot coverings) as required by CMS. Since 2009, operating rooms and procedure rooms must function under the same guidelines for sterility although endoscopic procedures are generally not considered sterile procedures. However, because of a number of outbreaks associated with endoscopy (such as hepatitis C), more stringent standards were imposed.

117. 2. A common age-related change in the stomach is decreased production of hydrochloric acid, which results in a slower digestive process. Motility slows and the stomach empties more slowly. The mucosal surface begins to atrophy and degenerate and other gastric acids and digestive enzymes decrease. As the person ages, these changes are likely to result in increased food intolerances and malabsorption (including decreased absorption of vitamin B-12).

118. 2. The flexible sigmoidoscope can examine a 45 to 50 cm/16 to 20 inches distance from the anus, compared to a rigid sigmoidoscope, which can examine only about 25 cm/20 inches. Additionally, the flexible sigmoidoscope allows video and still images to be obtained. The rigid sigmoidoscope is used much less frequently with the advent of flexible sigmoidoscopes although a rigid sigmoidoscope may be used along with a digital rectal exam for anal/rectal conditions.

119. 1. If during a gastroscopy a patient becomes very faint and light-headed and experiences hypotension, bradycardia, and diaphoresis, the most likely cause of these symptoms is a vasovagal response, which results from stimulation of baroreceptors during the procedure. The patient may briefly lose consciousness during the episode. The sudden drop in blood pressure decreases blood flow to the brain for a brief period. These episodes are usually transient but may be prolonged with depression of the central nervous system from sedation.

120. 3. If a patient has a hiatal hernia, important information to prevent symptoms (heartburn, reflux, dysphagia) includes eating small frequent meals and avoiding reclining for at least an hour after meals or eating within 2 hours of bedtime. The head of the patient's bed should be elevated on 4 to 8-inch blocks (pillows are not adequate). Medical treatments can include PPI and/or H2 blockers. Some patients may require surgical intervention if symptoms are severe.

121. 4. If a chemical spill occurs, the best initial resource to determine what actions to take is the Material Data Safety Sheet (MDSS), which must be on file for any chemicals in use. Spills are classified according to size:

- Small: ≤300 mL.
- Medium: >300 mL to 5L.
- Large: >5L.

Various kits are available to neutralize and absorb chemical spills. Large spills may require outside assistance. Some spills require alerts and evacuation because of noxious fumes or other risk factors while others require only restriction from the area of the spill to avoid contact.

122. 2. The primary purpose of a "time-out" period prior to beginning a procedure is to prevent surgical/procedural errors. Before a designated team member calls for the time out, all team members who will participate must be present and must communicate. The entire team must agree that they have the correct patient, correct site, and correct procedure. If a patient is to have more than one procedure or team members change, additional time-outs must be called before proceeding.

123. 4. The correct method of administration of vedolizumab (ENTYVIO®) is by infusion over 30 minutes. The drug comes packaged in a powdered form and must be reconstituted with 4.8 mL of sterile water injected into the vial, which is then swirled to mix for 15 seconds and allowed to sit for 20-30 minutes to dissolve. The vial is then inverted three times and 5 mL of solution withdrawn by sterile needle and syringe and injected into 250 mL of sterile 0.9% NaCl or Lactated Ringer's solution.

124. 3. If the nurse is to mix two medications for administration and injects air into vial A and then vial B, the next step is to withdraw the medication from vial B while the needle remains in the vial. Once the first medication is obtained, then the needle is inserted into vial A and that medication withdrawn. It is important that the vials are not contaminated with medication from the opposite vial. Prior to mixing medications, a compatibility chart should be accessed to ensure that the two medications can be mixed.

125. 1. Gastric aspirate, obtained per an NG tube, must be neutralized with bicarbonate within 30 minutes of collection. For this reason, it is often collected in a special tube that contains bicarbonate. If not, the sample (generally 1 mL but up to 5mL may be requested for suspected TB or fungal infections) must be transported to the laboratory immediately and the laboratory personnel alerted that the sample requires neutralization.

126. 3: Dumping syndrome usually responds to a change in dietary habits and is most often caused by carbohydrate intake, so increasing protein, reducing carbohydrates, and avoiding drinking fluids with meals may relieve symptoms. Acarbose is sometimes used with late-onset dumping syndrome (occurring 1 to 3 hours after eating) if other methods are ineffective. Octreotide requires injections and is used only for intractable symptoms because of adverse effects, such as diarrhea, distention, and cholelithiasis.

127. 2: A pH greater than 7 (alkaline) of aspirant from an NG tube most likely indicates that the tube tip is in the respiratory system. Gastric fluids tend to be acidic (although this can be altered by medications), so pH usually ranges from 1 to 4. The pH in intestinal fluids is less acidic and should be approximately 6 or higher. Some tubes have pH sensors in place and do not require aspiration to

check. Checking pH is not effective with continuous feedings because tube feedings usually have a pH of 6.6 and a neutralizing effect on gastrointestinal pH.

128. 4: The best time for scheduled evacuation is 20 to 30 minutes after a meal because eating stimulates motility. The scheduled time (usually daily but may be 3-4 times weekly depending on individual habits) should be at the same time each day, so work hours or activities should be considered. Stimulation may include drinking hot liquid or rectal stimulation (inserting a gloved, lubricated finger into the anus and running it around the rim of the sphincters). The best position for defecation is upright and leaning forward with knees elevated slightly. The patient should massage the abdomen, strain, and attempt to tighten abdominal muscles and relax sphincters if possible.

129. 2: Post-infectious irritable bowel syndrome is a chronic bowel inflammation that develops in some people after acute enteritis, characterized by altered bowel habits, usually with chronic diarrhea and abdominal pain. About two-thirds have predominately diarrhea, a fourth alternate between constipation and diarrhea, and the remaining have primarily constipation. Onset of symptoms is often abrupt. Symptoms often persist for years, with 40% still reporting symptoms after 6 years. Treatment usually entails antidiarrheal medication and a low fiber diet.

130. 3: Case control studies compare those with a condition (cases) to a group without it (controls) to determine if the affected group has characteristics that are different. Prospective cohort studies choose a group of patients without disease, assess risk factors, and then follow the group over time to determine (prospect for) which ones develop disease. Retrospective cohort studies are initiated after a condition develops and data is collected retrospectively from medical records to evaluate whether members of the cohort selected had exposure and developed disease. Cross-sectional studies assess both disease and exposure at the same time in a target population, evaluating the presence of disease at a point in time.

131. 1: Rectoceles can cause chronic constipation and difficulty in passing stool because of weakening of the muscles, contributing to fecal incontinence. Untreated, rectoceles can cause inflammation, ulcerations, and fistula formation. Pessaries may reduce the prolapse. Surgical repair may not correct all symptoms, especially underlying damage to muscles, and can result in surgical trauma to the rectum or sphincters, adding to the risk of incontinence. Rectoceles (rectal prolapses) occur when the muscles between the wall of the vagina and rectum weaken and the rectum prolapses or protrudes.

132. 4: A patient who has been stable on medications for gastric ulcer and begins to experience increasing back and epigastric pain that is unrelieved by medication may be experiencing erosion of the ulcer through the gastric serosa and into the surrounding organs and tissues, such as the pancreas or biliary tract. Penetration has a less acute presentation than perforation, which usually involves sudden acute abdominal pain (sometimes referred to the right shoulder), hypotension, bradycardia, omitting, and abdominal distention and rigidity.

133. 1: Peristomal abscess is common with active Crohn's disease distal to the stoma. Crohn's disease is a form of inflammatory bowel disease in which ulcerations occur in the small and sometimes the large intestines. Peristomal abscess is characterized by open (from fistulae) and closed lesions that are painful, swollen, and erythematous. Peristomal abscess may also occur after stomal revision because of contamination from skin bacteria. Colostomy irrigation may result in perforation that causes abscess formation. A peristomal abscess rarely heals spontaneously but requires surgical incision.

134. 3: Cimetidine (brand name Tagamet): First developed but used less frequently than others because of inhibition of enzymes that results in drug interactions, especially with contraceptive agents and estrogen. Ranitidine (brand name Zantac): Developed to decrease drug interactions and improve patient tolerance. Its activity is about 10 times that of cimetidine. It may be used in combination with other drugs to treat ulcers. Famotidine (brand name Pepcid): May be combined with an antacid to increase the speed of effects, as it has a slow onset. It may be used pre-surgically to reduce postoperative nausea. Nizatidine (brand name Axid): Latest to be developed and about equal in potency and action to ranitidine.

135. 4: Anal manometry measures the pressure of the sphincter muscles, the degree of sensation in the rectum, and whether the neural reflexes that control normal bowel movements are intact. Anal wink (anocutaneous reflex, a reflexive contraction of the anus in response to gentle stroking or stimulation of the skin around the rectum) and Bulbocavernosus reflex (a reflexive contraction of the anus in response to natural or electrical stimulation of the bulbocavernosus muscle of the penis), are used to determine interruption or defect in the reflex arc. Endoanal ultrasound is used to diagnose perianal fistulas and abscesses and to assess sphincter damage.

136. 1: Improving staff communication includes ensuring that the appropriate staff person receives laboratory test results on time and establishing a process for taking orders/report and read back for verbal/telephone orders. Other provisions include:

- Identifying patients correctly: 2 identifiers for medicines, blood, or blood products.
- Using medications safely: complete medicine list, label medications, removing concentrated electrolytes from patient care units.
- Preventing infection: CDC handwashing procedures, infection control guidelines.
- Identifying safety risk: includes fall prevention.
- Preventing surgical mistakes: checklists, marking surgical site, presurgical pause.

137. 2: Anal sphincter electromyography (EMG) assesses muscle contractions to determine if the sphincter muscles are contracting properly. Drugs such as muscle relaxants and cholinergic and anti-cholinergic preparations can affect the outcome of the test. The procedure begins with the patient lying on the left side. A small lubricated sponge or plug electrode is inserted into the anal canal. Alternately, needle electrodes may be used. The patient must lie still during the procedure or results will be affected. Electrical activity of the anal sphincter muscles is recorded on a computer screen while the patient tightens the sphincter muscles, relaxes, and pushes.

138. 4: Monitoring intake and output is most important in preventing fluid and electrolyte imbalance along with ensuring adequate nutrition. During episodes of diarrhea, the patient should substitute water with a sports drink designed to replenish electrolytes and supply nutrition. With electrolyte imbalance, just increasing the oral intake of fluids is not sufficient because these fluids will be excreted through the kidneys and may not correct the electrolyte imbalance. If stools are too liquid, the patient can increase fiber: and if stools are too dry, sodium. Antidiarrheal agents should not be taken routinely but as necessary when dietary changes are insufficient.

139. 2: While some anal mucous discharge is normal, copious discharge is often associated with diversion colitis in which the distal segment becomes inflamed. Treatment includes rectal irrigation and topical steroids as well as oral antibiotics. The perianal area should be cleansed. Applying protective cream or ointment prevents irritation of the skin. The mucous fistula should be checked each time the appliance is changed and mucous gently wiped from the opening. The stoma should remain pink. Changes in color or swelling may indicate compromised circulation or infection.

140. 1: Under the ANA Nursing Code of Ethics, autonomy and self-determination are viewed within the broad context of diverse cultures. The idea of individualism is less important in some cultures, so the nurse must respect and appreciate the patient's right to be guided by her family. Trying to convince the patient to assert herself may just lead to emotional conflict. This is not an appropriate concern for the ethics committee, because the woman is not being forced to comply with family decisions but chooses to do so.

141. 3: Kinesthetic learners learn best by handling, doing, and practicing and should be allowed to handle supplies/equipment with minimal directions. They benefit from demonstrating their understanding by doing the procedure. Visual learners learn best by seeing and reading and benefit from written directions, videos, diagrams, pictures, and demonstrations. Auditory learners learn best by listening and talking, so procedures should be explained during demonstrations. Auditory learners benefit from audiotapes and extra time for questions.

142. 4: Patients who receive multiple transfusions with citrated blood products must be carefully monitored for hypocalcemia. Calcium is important for transmitting nerve impulses and regulating muscle contraction and relaxation, including the myocardium. Calcium activates enzymes that stimulate chemical reactions and has a role in coagulation of blood. Values include:

- Normal values: 8.2 to 10.2 mg/dL
- Hypocalcemia: less than 8.2 mg/dL
- Critical value: less than 7 mg/dL
- Hypercalcemia: greater than 10.2 mg/dL
- Critical value: greater than 12 mg/dL

Symptoms include tetany, tingling, seizures, altered mental status, and ventricular tachycardia. Treatment is calcium replacement and vitamin D.

143. 2: The PEG tube does not have an inflatable balloon, but the tube should be stabilized by pulling gently to ensure the internal bumper is against the abdominal wall and then sliding the external stabilizer to 1.5 cm above skin. Replacing the PEG tube is done only if the leakage cannot be otherwise controlled. Routine skin care, including application of barrier ointment or other skin sealant, is necessary to prevent skin breakdown. In some cases, alginates, foam dressing, gauze, or pouching may be necessary.

144. 1: A positive Murphy's sign is indicative of cholecystitis but is negative with choledocholithiasis and ascending cholangitis. This test is not accurate for geriatric patients, so a negative finding does not rule out cholecystitis for these patients. To test for Murphy's sign, hook the fingers under the right costal margin at the midpoint, palpating deeply, and ask the patient to inhale deeply. Positive results occur with pain causing the patient to stop inspiring. The Rovsing's sign—pain in the RLQ when left-sided abdominal pressure is applied—suggests appendicitis along with RLQ pain (rebound tenderness) on quick removal of pressure.

145. 2: Esophageal diverticulum is a contraindication for upper GI endoscopy because the scope may enter the diverticulum sac, resulting in a perforation. Endoscopy is indicated for complicated reflux disease, such as when the patient exhibits dysphagia or iron deficiency anemia and is routinely used to diagnose, biopsy tissue, assess, and treat Barrett's esophagus. Endoscopy is usually done within 24 hours after caustic esophageal injuries, such as from accidental or deliberate ingestion of liquid or crystalline alkali, to assess the degree of mucosal tissue damage.

146. 4: While trends will show some normal variation, if the trend becomes erratic and measures are inconsistent, this suggests that the processes of care are not consistent or are inadequate. Tracking and trending is central to developing research-supported, evidence-based practice and is part of continuous quality improvement. Once processes and outcomes measurements are selected, then at least one measure should be tracked for a number of periods of time, usually in increments of 4 weeks or quarterly. This tracking can be used to present graphical representation of results that will show trends.

147. 1: While all of these are important, studies have shown that completing a safety pre-procedure checklist is highly effective in reducing infections and other complications. Checklists should be standardized according to discipline/procedure and required for all procedures to ensure that infection control and safety practices are followed. Checklists usually include ensuring correct patient, following the correct procedure, and checking patient records to make sure orders have been carried out. Checklists vary but may include handwashing, use of barrier precautions, and checking for known allergies.

148. 3: A visit from a recovered ostomate who is functioning well can provide invaluable support. Refusing to look at the stoma or participate in care after surgery is very common as patients grapple with the alteration in body image and anxiety about their role in the family and society, their sexuality, and their ability to resume their normal activities. Family members should be encouraged to learn about ostomy care and to provide support as well, but they may also be very stressed and unsure. Referral to a psychologist may be indicated if the patient cannot overcome her anxiety and fears.

149. 2: Over-transfusing to treat esophageal variceal hemorrhage can result in increased central and portal venous pressures, increasing the risk of rebleeding, so the patient must be monitored very carefully. Coagulopathy is commonly found related to underlying cirrhosis. If actively bleeding, those with an INR above 1.8 to 2.0 or with platelet counts below 50,000 should be treated with fresh frozen plasma (20 mL/kg loading, followed by 10 mg/kg every 6 hours) or platelets. About half the hemorrhages will stop spontaneously, but over half of these patients experience rebleeding within 7 days.

150. 3: A decrease in hematocrit greater than 10% within 48 hours of hospital admission is predictive of severe pancreatitis. Other warning signs include a BUN greater than 5 mg/dL, serum calcium less than 8 mg/dl, a base deficit greater than 4 mEq/L, PO_2 less than 60 mm Hg, and fluid retention/sequestration greater than 6 liters. On admission, indications include age over 55 years, white blood count greater than 16,000, serum glucose greater than 200 mg/dL, serum LDH >350 IU/L, and Aspartate aminotransferase (AST) greater than 250 U/mL.

151. 2:

1. Standard I, Quality of Practice: Collecting data and participating in quality of care activities.
2. Professional Practice Evaluation: Participating in performance appraisal, feedback, peer review, and demonstrating cultural competency.
3. Education: Having commitment to lifelong learning.
4. Collegiality: Sharing with others, mentoring, participating in professional organizations.
5. Ethics: Complying with ANA Code of Ethics, maintaining privacy and protecting patient autonomy.
6. Collaboration: Collaborating with other health professionals, patient, and family members.
7. Research: Participating in research, reading, and utilizing research.

8. Resource Utilization: Considering costs, effectiveness, and safety, and delegating care.
9. Leader: Utilizing teamwork and mentoring and promoting the profession.

152. 1: The first method to use to clear a blockage in one of the endoscopic channels is to flush with water using a small syringe (1 to 5 mL). A small syringe applies more water pressure than a larger syringe, although the larger syringe is better for suctioning. Water also applies more pressure than flushing with air and is better able to remove residue that may be blocking the channel. Only if flushing is ineffective should the tube be removed and wire used to cleanse residue. Scrupulous cleaning after use helps to avoid blockage.

153. 2: Proton pump inhibitors and antibiotics may interfere with the results of both the urea breath test and the fecal antigen assay for *H. pylori*, so PPIs should be discontinued 1 to 2 weeks prior to testing and antibiotics at least 4 weeks prior. If patients cannot discontinue the medications, then serologic ELISA testing may be done, but it has only 80% accuracy compared to 95% accuracy for the breath and fecal tests. Endoscopic testing is usually not recommended for diagnosis, although, if done for other reasons, gastric biopsies may be taken to rule out or diagnose *H. pylori*.

154. 3: A low-fat diet is usually recommended for those with chronic pancreatitis. Because production of pancreatic enzymes may be impaired, patients may also need to take pancreatic enzymes with meals. If insulin production is affected, then some may require treatment for diabetes with insulin and diet modified to restrict carbohydrates. Since about 45% of those with chronic pancreatitis suffer from alcohol abuse, restricting alcohol intake is critical, so some patients may require referral to substance abuse programs.

155. 1: A patient who has had percutaneous transhepatic cholangiography is most at risk for bleeding, peritonitis, and septicemia. During the procedure, a flexible needle is inserted into the liver, increasing risk of bleeding, in order to aspirate bile. A water-soluble contrast agent is injected, the fluoroscopy table tilted, and multiple x-rays taken. Aspirating as much contrast agent and bile as possible prior to removing the needle helps to reduce the risk of peritonitis. Antibiotics should be administered to reduce incidence of septicemia.

156. 4: The primary purpose of a TIPS is to reduce portal hypertension by treating ascites. A cannula is threaded through the jugular vein to the portal vein and an expandable stent inserted to shunt fluid between the hepatic vein and portal circulation. TIPS is indicated for ascites that does not respond to more conservative treatments and helps to reduce sodium retention so that diuretics can act more effectively. Patients who will be referred for liver transplantation often have a TIPS while awaiting an organ.

157. 2: Applying a heating pad to the right shoulder or scapula area after laparoscopic cholecystectomy for 15 to 20 minutes each hour may help to reduce pain caused by migration of carbon dioxide used for insufflation during the surgical procedure. Pain is usually not severe, so opioids are rarely indicated. Complications are rare, and this procedure is often done on an outpatient basis, but patients should be advised to report vomiting, loss of appetite, increasing pain, temperature, and abdominal distention.

158. 3: After cholecystectomy, patients who had experienced preoperative fat intolerance should begin to add fat back into the diet in small increments to allow the body to adjust. In some cases, the liver may not produce enough bile to metabolize a high intake of fat and some fat restriction (40 to 50 g daily) may be indicated. Generally, patients are able to resume eating a normal diet shortly

after surgery and should not exhibit signs of dietary intolerance, such as pain, distention, nausea, or vomiting.

159. 4: Fecal occult blood—yearly: checks for blood in stool. Screening at age 50 with average risk and age 40 with increased risk:

- Flexible sigmoidoscopy—every 5 years: scope to check for polyps or signs of cancer in rectum and lower third of colon. (Often done with fecal occult blood test.)
- Colonoscopy—every 10 years or as follow-up for abnormalities in other screening: longer flexible scope, usually with anesthesia, to check rectum and entire colon, remove polyps, do biopsies, and provide surveillance of inflammatory bowel disease.
- Double contrast barium enema—every 5 years: S-ray with contrast to visualize intestinal abnormalities.

160. 3: A nasoenteric tube for an adult should be marked prior to insertion with measurements including the distance from nose to earlobe, plus earlobe to xiphoid process, plus 8 to 10 inches for enteric placement. Six inches are needed for gastric placement. The nasoenteric tube tip is initially placed in the stomach (verified by chest x-ray) and then moves into the small intestine through peristalsis over about 24 hours. Proper placement should be reconfirmed before every feeding by checking tube length measurement, aspirating and observing aspirant, and checking pH.

161. 2: Following bariatric surgery, such as the lap band procedure, general guidelines advise limiting total meal intake to less than one cup, with 3 meals daily (containing protein and fiber) and two protein snacks. Patients should be advised to chew slowly and thoroughly and to eat nutrient-rich foods, but should avoid combining food and liquids. Liquids should be taken 90 minutes after meals and up to 15 minutes prior to a meal, but caloric liquids (such as alcoholic beverages and juices) should be avoided.

162. 1: Hemolytic uremic syndrome (HUS) is the most serious complication of enteritis caused by *E. coli,* such as type O157:H7. Children under 5 and the elderly are especially at risk. HUS is characterized by microangiopathic hemolytic anemia, thrombocytopenia, and renal failure. HUS may affect the neurological system, resulting in seizures, stroke, and coma. About half of those who survive HUS will develop chronic renal problems. Various organs, such as the heart and brain, may be affected because HUS damages the blood vessels and causes clots to form in capillaries and arterioles.

163. 4: These symptoms are indicative of intestinal obstruction, which may be partial or complete. Obstructions are common because strictures develop in the bowel from repeated ulcerations of mucoid tissue. Chronic diarrhea is common, and some diarrhea may persist even with obstruction, depending on the location and degree of obstruction. Other common complications include abscesses, fistulas (especially from the small bowel to the skin), fissures, and malnutrition. Lesions associated with Crohn's disease are most common in the distal ileum and ascending colon.

164. 2: Total parenteral nutrition (TPN) is high in glucose, so patients should have blood glucose levels monitored every 6 hours to evaluate hyperglycemia. Some patients may require insulin during administration of parenteral nutrition. Symptoms of hyperglycemia may include increased thirst, increased urination, blurred vision, and lethargy. Some patients may experience a rebound hypoglycemia when TPN is discontinued. The goal of TPN is usually for the patient to gain about 0.5 kg daily. Once the patient's symptoms decrease and weight stabilizes, the patient is placed on oral elemental feedings.

165. 3: The most effective method for monitoring small changes in abdominal ascitic fluid is daily measuring of abdominal girth and weighing. This should be done routinely to assess the effectiveness of treatment. A large fluid accumulation may be indicated by bulging flanks with the patient in supine position. Abdominal percussion may also identify ascites, but assessing small increases or decreases is difficult. An abdominal fluid wave is usually not noted until there is a large accumulation of fluid.

166. 3: A permanent colostomy in the descending colon is most likely to result in semi-soft, mushy stool. A colostomy in the ascending colon results in liquid stool, as little absorption has taken place as liquid stool enters the colon from the small intestine. A transverse colostomy results in semi-liquid, somewhat mushy stool. Because the sigmoid colostomy is directly above the rectum, most excess fluid has been absorbed by the proximal colon, so stool tends to be solid.

167. 4: Upon completion of an endoscopic procedure, before the endoscope is removed from the procedure room and taken to the cleaning area, using standard precautions the exterior should be wiped down with a gauze pad to remove discharge and debris (feces, mucus, blood) and then the suction channel and water channel flushed with water until the water runs clear. Once in the cleaning area, procedures will vary depending on whether manual cleaning is completed or automated but usually begin with leak testing and cleaning and flushing with enzymatic detergent prior to placing in high-level disinfectant.

168. 2: Diabetic patients who are well controlled on insulin are usually advised to take half of their usual dosage on the morning of a scheduled endoscopic procedure. Diabetics who take oral medications to control diabetes should omit the dosage for that morning. Glucose levels should be monitored when the patient arrives for the procedure and the physician notified if the patient is hypoglycemic (<60 mg/dL) or hyperglycemic (>200 mg/dL). IV solutions administered may depend on blood glucose level. Those who are hypoglycemic may receive 50% glucose solution, and those who are hyperglycemic, NS.

169. 1: Patients undergoing sigmoidoscopy (rigid or flexible) usually require no or minimal sedation, although patients with low pain threshold or severe anxiety may need moderate/conscious sedation. Moderate sedation (a narcotic such as fentanyl and a benzodiazepine such as midazolam) is usually indicated for endoscopic procedures, such as upper endoscopy and colonoscopy. Procedures that are complicated or prolonged, such as ECRP, may require deep sedation with the same drugs as well as droperidol or propofol. General anesthesia is generally indicated only for complex and surgical procedures because of increased risks associated with general anesthesia.

170. 3: The best method to verify placement of a small-bore NG tube is with a chest x-ray. While aspirating fluid may indicate gastric placement, the tip may be in the esophagus. A gastric fluid pH less than 4 usually indicates that the tube is in the stomach, but some medications, such as proton pump inhibitors, may alter pH. Injecting air and auscultating may be inaccurate because the air sounds in the bronchial tree sound similar, and NG tubes can easily enter the trachea and a bronchus. Misplacement into the bronchus may not be evident on abdominal x-ray.

171. 3: Flumazenil is a reversal agent for benzodiazepines, such as midazolam and diazepam. Flumazenil is usually given in a dose of 0.2 mg over 15 seconds and can be repeated every minute to a total of 1 mg and then at 30 minute to 60 minute intervals because the action of flumazenil is shorter than that of benzodiazepines. Therefore, patients must be monitored for at least 2 hours after administration to determine if further dosage is required. Naloxone should also be available as a reversal agent for opioids, such as fentanyl and meperidine.

172. 4: The best positioning for a paracentesis is for the patient to sit upright on a chair or on the side of the bed because this causes the fluid to accumulate in the lower and anterior abdomen, making drainage more effective. Patients who are confined to bed may be placed in the Fowler's position. Fluid should drain by gravity. The patient must be carefully monitored and VS taken frequently as vascular collapse/hypovolemia may occur as the body compensates for the fluid loss by shifting fluid from the vascular system to the peritoneal cavity.

173. 1: The method that is the most successful for postpyloric placement of enteral feeding tubes is to inject about 350 mL of air and place the patient on the right side. An alternate method is to administer the prokinetic metoclopramide to stimulate peristalsis and then to position the patient on the right side. Combining both methods is not indicated. The air insufflation method usually results in faster placement, especially if the patient has received opioids, which tend to slow peristalsis.

174. 4: During an upper GI endoscopy procedure, it's important to aggressively suction all accumulated saliva and emesis to prevent aspiration. Pre-medicating with an antiemetic is usually not recommended, and positioning of the patient may have little effect. Recommendations for NPO status prior to endoscopic procedures vary slightly from 6 hours to 8 hours to ensure the stomach has emptied. While the endoscopic procedure may induce vomiting, 12 hours of NPO status is more than required.

175. 1: Patients have a right to refuse treatment for religious or other personal reasons, so the most appropriate action is to simply provide the patient with factual information about the disease, treatments, and prognosis in a neutral manner, without trying to coerce or frighten the patient. In some cases, patients may change their minds when presented with information, but the nurse should remain supportive regardless of the patient's decision. Asking the family to intervene is not appropriate and refusal of treatment alone does not suggest the need for referral to a psychologist.

How to Overcome Test Anxiety

Just the thought of taking a test is enough to make most people a little nervous. A test is an important event that can have a long-term impact on your future, so it's important to take it seriously and it's natural to feel anxious about performing well. But just because anxiety is normal, that doesn't mean that it's helpful in test taking, or that you should simply accept it as part of your life. Anxiety can have a variety of effects. These effects can be mild, like making you feel slightly nervous, or severe, like blocking your ability to focus or remember even a simple detail.

If you experience test anxiety—whether severe or mild—it's important to know how to beat it. To discover this, first you need to understand what causes test anxiety.

Causes of Test Anxiety

While we often think of anxiety as an uncontrollable emotional state, it can actually be caused by simple, practical things. One of the most common causes of test anxiety is that a person does not feel adequately prepared for their test. This feeling can be the result of many different issues such as poor study habits or lack of organization, but the most common culprit is time management. Starting to study too late, failing to organize your study time to cover all of the material, or being distracted while you study will mean that you're not well prepared for the test. This may lead to cramming the night before, which will cause you to be physically and mentally exhausted for the test. Poor time management also contributes to feelings of stress, fear, and hopelessness as you realize you are not well prepared but don't know what to do about it.

Other times, test anxiety is not related to your preparation for the test but comes from unresolved fear. This may be a past failure on a test, or poor performance on tests in general. It may come from comparing yourself to others who seem to be performing better or from the stress of living up to expectations. Anxiety may be driven by fears of the future—how failure on this test would affect your educational and career goals. These fears are often completely irrational, but they can still negatively impact your test performance.

> **Review Video: 3 Reasons You Have Test Anxiety**
> Visit mometrix.com/academy and enter code: 428468

Elements of Test Anxiety

As mentioned earlier, test anxiety is considered to be an emotional state, but it has physical and mental components as well. Sometimes you may not even realize that you are suffering from test anxiety until you notice the physical symptoms. These can include trembling hands, rapid heartbeat, sweating, nausea, and tense muscles. Extreme anxiety may lead to fainting or vomiting. Obviously, any of these symptoms can have a negative impact on testing. It is important to recognize them as soon as they begin to occur so that you can address the problem before it damages your performance.

> **Review Video: 3 Ways to Tell You Have Test Anxiety**
> Visit mometrix.com/academy and enter code: 927847

The mental components of test anxiety include trouble focusing and inability to remember learned information. During a test, your mind is on high alert, which can help you recall information and stay focused for an extended period of time. However, anxiety interferes with your mind's natural processes, causing you to blank out, even on the questions you know well. The strain of testing during anxiety makes it difficult to stay focused, especially on a test that may take several hours. Extreme anxiety can take a huge mental toll, making it difficult not only to recall test information but even to understand the test questions or pull your thoughts together.

> **Review Video: How Test Anxiety Affects Memory**
> Visit mometrix.com/academy and enter code: 609003

Effects of Test Anxiety

Test anxiety is like a disease—if left untreated, it will get progressively worse. Anxiety leads to poor performance, and this reinforces the feelings of fear and failure, which in turn lead to poor performances on subsequent tests. It can grow from a mild nervousness to a crippling condition. If allowed to progress, test anxiety can have a big impact on your schooling, and consequently on your future.

Test anxiety can spread to other parts of your life. Anxiety on tests can become anxiety in any stressful situation, and blanking on a test can turn into panicking in a job situation. But fortunately, you don't have to let anxiety rule your testing and determine your grades. There are a number of relatively simple steps you can take to move past anxiety and function normally on a test and in the rest of life.

> **Review Video: How Test Anxiety Impacts Your Grades**
> Visit mometrix.com/academy and enter code: 939819

Physical Steps for Beating Test Anxiety

While test anxiety is a serious problem, the good news is that it can be overcome. It doesn't have to control your ability to think and remember information. While it may take time, you can begin taking steps today to beat anxiety.

Just as your first hint that you may be struggling with anxiety comes from the physical symptoms, the first step to treating it is also physical. Rest is crucial for having a clear, strong mind. If you are tired, it is much easier to give in to anxiety. But if you establish good sleep habits, your body and mind will be ready to perform optimally, without the strain of exhaustion. Additionally, sleeping well helps you to retain information better, so you're more likely to recall the answers when you see the test questions.

Getting good sleep means more than going to bed on time. It's important to allow your brain time to relax. Take study breaks from time to time so it doesn't get overworked, and don't study right before bed. Take time to rest your mind before trying to rest your body, or you may find it difficult to fall asleep.

Review Video: The Importance of Sleep for Your Brain
Visit mometrix.com/academy and enter code: 319338

Along with sleep, other aspects of physical health are important in preparing for a test. Good nutrition is vital for good brain function. Sugary foods and drinks may give a burst of energy but this burst is followed by a crash, both physically and emotionally. Instead, fuel your body with protein and vitamin-rich foods.

Also, drink plenty of water. Dehydration can lead to headaches and exhaustion, especially if your brain is already under stress from the rigors of the test. Particularly if your test is a long one, drink water during the breaks. And if possible, take an energy-boosting snack to eat between sections.

Review Video: How Diet Can Affect your Mood
Visit mometrix.com/academy and enter code: 624317

Along with sleep and diet, a third important part of physical health is exercise. Maintaining a steady workout schedule is helpful, but even taking 5-minute study breaks to walk can help get your blood pumping faster and clear your head. Exercise also releases endorphins, which contribute to a positive feeling and can help combat test anxiety.

When you nurture your physical health, you are also contributing to your mental health. If your body is healthy, your mind is much more likely to be healthy as well. So take time to rest, nourish your body with healthy food and water, and get moving as much as possible. Taking these physical steps will make you stronger and more able to take the mental steps necessary to overcome test anxiety.

Review Video: How to Stay Healthy and Prevent Test Anxiety
Visit mometrix.com/academy and enter code: 877894

Mental Steps for Beating Test Anxiety

Working on the mental side of test anxiety can be more challenging, but as with the physical side, there are clear steps you can take to overcome it. As mentioned earlier, test anxiety often stems from lack of preparation, so the obvious solution is to prepare for the test. Effective studying may be the most important weapon you have for beating test anxiety, but you can and should employ several other mental tools to combat fear.

First, boost your confidence by reminding yourself of past success—tests or projects that you aced. If you're putting as much effort into preparing for this test as you did for those, there's no reason you should expect to fail here. Work hard to prepare; then trust your preparation.

Second, surround yourself with encouraging people. It can be helpful to find a study group, but be sure that the people you're around will encourage a positive attitude. If you spend time with others who are anxious or cynical, this will only contribute to your own anxiety. Look for others who are motivated to study hard from a desire to succeed, not from a fear of failure.

Third, reward yourself. A test is physically and mentally tiring, even without anxiety, and it can be helpful to have something to look forward to. Plan an activity following the test, regardless of the outcome, such as going to a movie or getting ice cream.

When you are taking the test, if you find yourself beginning to feel anxious, remind yourself that you know the material. Visualize successfully completing the test. Then take a few deep, relaxing breaths and return to it. Work through the questions carefully but with confidence, knowing that you are capable of succeeding.

Developing a healthy mental approach to test taking will also aid in other areas of life. Test anxiety affects more than just the actual test—it can be damaging to your mental health and even contribute to depression. It's important to beat test anxiety before it becomes a problem for more than testing.

> **Review Video: Test Anxiety and Depression**
> Visit mometrix.com/academy and enter code: 904704

Study Strategy

Being prepared for the test is necessary to combat anxiety, but what does being prepared look like? You may study for hours on end and still not feel prepared. What you need is a strategy for test prep. The next few pages outline our recommended steps to help you plan out and conquer the challenge of preparation.

Step 1: Scope Out the Test

Learn everything you can about the format (multiple choice, essay, etc.) and what will be on the test. Gather any study materials, course outlines, or sample exams that may be available. Not only will this help you to prepare, but knowing what to expect can help to alleviate test anxiety.

Step 2: Map Out the Material

Look through the textbook or study guide and make note of how many chapters or sections it has. Then divide these over the time you have. For example, if a book has 15 chapters and you have five days to study, you need to cover three chapters each day. Even better, if you have the time, leave an extra day at the end for overall review after you have gone through the material in depth.

If time is limited, you may need to prioritize the material. Look through it and make note of which sections you think you already have a good grasp on, and which need review. While you are studying, skim quickly through the familiar sections and take more time on the challenging parts. Write out your plan so you don't get lost as you go. Having a written plan also helps you feel more in control of the study, so anxiety is less likely to arise from feeling overwhelmed at the amount to cover. A sample plan may look like this:

- Day 1: Skim chapters 1–4, study chapter 5 (especially pages 31–33)
- Day 2: Study chapters 6–7, skim chapters 8–9
- Day 3: Skim chapter 10, study chapters 11–12 (especially pages 87–90)
- Day 4: Study chapters 13–15
- Day 5: Overall review (focus most on chapters 5, 6, and 12), take practice test

Step 3: Gather Your Tools

Decide what study method works best for you. Do you prefer to highlight in the book as you study and then go back over the highlighted portions? Or do you type out notes of the important information? Or is it helpful to make flashcards that you can carry with you? Assemble the pens, index cards, highlighters, post-it notes, and any other materials you may need so you won't be distracted by getting up to find things while you study.

If you're having a hard time retaining the information or organizing your notes, experiment with different methods. For example, try color-coding by subject with colored pens, highlighters, or post-it notes. If you learn better by hearing, try recording yourself reading your notes so you can listen while in the car, working out, or simply sitting at your desk. Ask a friend to quiz you from your flashcards, or try teaching someone the material to solidify it in your mind.

Step 4: Create Your Environment

It's important to avoid distractions while you study. This includes both the obvious distractions like visitors and the subtle distractions like an uncomfortable chair (or a too-comfortable couch that makes you want to fall asleep). Set up the best study environment possible: good lighting and a comfortable work area. If background music helps you focus, you may want to turn it on, but otherwise keep the room quiet. If you are using a computer to take notes, be sure you don't have any other windows open, especially applications like social media, games, or anything else that could distract you. Silence your phone and turn off notifications. Be sure to keep water close by so you stay hydrated while you study (but avoid unhealthy drinks and snacks).

Also, take into account the best time of day to study. Are you freshest first thing in the morning? Try to set aside some time then to work through the material. Is your mind clearer in the afternoon or evening? Schedule your study session then. Another method is to study at the same time of day that you will take the test, so that your brain gets used to working on the material at that time and will be ready to focus at test time.

Step 5: Study!

Once you have done all the study preparation, it's time to settle into the actual studying. Sit down, take a few moments to settle your mind so you can focus, and begin to follow your study plan. Don't give in to distractions or let yourself procrastinate. This is your time to prepare so you'll be ready to fearlessly approach the test. Make the most of the time and stay focused.

Of course, you don't want to burn out. If you study too long you may find that you're not retaining the information very well. Take regular study breaks. For example, taking five minutes out of every hour to walk briskly, breathing deeply and swinging your arms, can help your mind stay fresh.

As you get to the end of each chapter or section, it's a good idea to do a quick review. Remind yourself of what you learned and work on any difficult parts. When you feel that you've mastered the material, move on to the next part. At the end of your study session, briefly skim through your notes again.

But while review is helpful, cramming last minute is NOT. If at all possible, work ahead so that you won't need to fit all your study into the last day. Cramming overloads your brain with more information than it can process and retain, and your tired mind may struggle to recall even previously learned information when it is overwhelmed with last-minute study. Also, the urgent nature of cramming and the stress placed on your brain contribute to anxiety. You'll be more likely to go to the test feeling unprepared and having trouble thinking clearly.

So don't cram, and don't stay up late before the test, even just to review your notes at a leisurely pace. Your brain needs rest more than it needs to go over the information again. In fact, plan to finish your studies by noon or early afternoon the day before the test. Give your brain the rest of the day to relax or focus on other things, and get a good night's sleep. Then you will be fresh for the test and better able to recall what you've studied.

Step 6: Take a practice test

Many courses offer sample tests, either online or in the study materials. This is an excellent resource to check whether you have mastered the material, as well as to prepare for the test format and environment.

Check the test format ahead of time: the number of questions, the type (multiple choice, free response, etc.), and the time limit. Then create a plan for working through them. For example, if you have 30 minutes to take a 60-question test, your limit is 30 seconds per question. Spend less time on the questions you know well so that you can take more time on the difficult ones.

If you have time to take several practice tests, take the first one open book, with no time limit. Work through the questions at your own pace and make sure you fully understand them. Gradually work up to taking a test under test conditions: sit at a desk with all study materials put away and set a timer. Pace yourself to make sure you finish the test with time to spare and go back to check your answers if you have time.

After each test, check your answers. On the questions you missed, be sure you understand why you missed them. Did you misread the question (tests can use tricky wording)? Did you forget the information? Or was it something you hadn't learned? Go back and study any shaky areas that the practice tests reveal.

Taking these tests not only helps with your grade, but also aids in combating test anxiety. If you're already used to the test conditions, you're less likely to worry about it, and working through tests until you're scoring well gives you a confidence boost. Go through the practice tests until you feel comfortable, and then you can go into the test knowing that you're ready for it.

Test Tips

On test day, you should be confident, knowing that you've prepared well and are ready to answer the questions. But aside from preparation, there are several test day strategies you can employ to maximize your performance.

First, as stated before, get a good night's sleep the night before the test (and for several nights before that, if possible). Go into the test with a fresh, alert mind rather than staying up late to study.

Try not to change too much about your normal routine on the day of the test. It's important to eat a nutritious breakfast, but if you normally don't eat breakfast at all, consider eating just a protein bar. If you're a coffee drinker, go ahead and have your normal coffee. Just make sure you time it so that the caffeine doesn't wear off right in the middle of your test. Avoid sugary beverages, and drink enough water to stay hydrated but not so much that you need a restroom break 10 minutes into the test. If your test isn't first thing in the morning, consider going for a walk or doing a light workout before the test to get your blood flowing.

Allow yourself enough time to get ready, and leave for the test with plenty of time to spare so you won't have the anxiety of scrambling to arrive in time. Another reason to be early is to select a good seat. It's helpful to sit away from doors and windows, which can be distracting. Find a good seat, get out your supplies, and settle your mind before the test begins.

When the test begins, start by going over the instructions carefully, even if you already know what to expect. Make sure you avoid any careless mistakes by following the directions.

Then begin working through the questions, pacing yourself as you've practiced. If you're not sure on an answer, don't spend too much time on it, and don't let it shake your confidence. Either skip it and come back later, or eliminate as many wrong answers as possible and guess among the remaining ones. Don't dwell on these questions as you continue—put them out of your mind and focus on what lies ahead.

Be sure to read all of the answer choices, even if you're sure the first one is the right answer. Sometimes you'll find a better one if you keep reading. But don't second-guess yourself if you do immediately know the answer. Your gut instinct is usually right. Don't let test anxiety rob you of the information you know.

If you have time at the end of the test (and if the test format allows), go back and review your answers. Be cautious about changing any, since your first instinct tends to be correct, but make sure you didn't misread any of the questions or accidentally mark the wrong answer choice. Look over any you skipped and make an educated guess.

At the end, leave the test feeling confident. You've done your best, so don't waste time worrying about your performance or wishing you could change anything. Instead, celebrate the successful completion of this test. And finally, use this test to learn how to deal with anxiety even better next time.

> **Review Video: 5 Tips to Beat Test Anxiety**
> Visit mometrix.com/academy and enter code: 570656

Important Qualification

Not all anxiety is created equal. If your test anxiety is causing major issues in your life beyond the classroom or testing center, or if you are experiencing troubling physical symptoms related to your anxiety, it may be a sign of a serious physiological or psychological condition. If this sounds like your situation, we strongly encourage you to seek professional help.

Thank You

We at Mometrix would like to extend our heartfelt thanks to you, our friend and patron, for allowing us to play a part in your journey. It is a privilege to serve people from all walks of life who are unified in their commitment to building the best future they can for themselves.

The preparation you devote to these important testing milestones may be the most valuable educational opportunity you have for making a real difference in your life. We encourage you to put your heart into it—that feeling of succeeding, overcoming, and yes, conquering will be well worth the hours you've invested.

We want to hear your story, your struggles and your successes, and if you see any opportunities for us to improve our materials so we can help others even more effectively in the future, please share that with us as well. **The team at Mometrix would be absolutely thrilled to hear from you!** So please, send us an email (support@mometrix.com) and let's stay in touch.

If you'd like some additional help, check out these other resources we offer for your exam:

http://mometrixflashcards.com/CGRN

Additional Bonus Material

Due to our efforts to try to keep this book to a manageable length, we've created a link that will give you access to all of your additional bonus material.

Please visit https://www.mometrix.com/bonus948/cgrn to access the information.